Heartbeat

HEARTBEAT

A Practical Guide to Lifelong Heart Health for You and Your Family

DR AMIT BHUSHAN SHARMA
and
AMBIKA RIKHYE

Foreword by Boman Irani

BLOOMSBURY
NEW DELHI • LONDON • OXFORD • NEW YORK • SYDNEY

BLOOMSBURY INDIA
Bloomsbury Publishing India Pvt. Ltd
Second Floor, LSC Building No. 4, DDA Complex, Pocket C – 6 & 7,
Vasant Kunj, New Delhi, 110070

BLOOMSBURY, BLOOMSBURY INDIA and the Diana logo
are trademarks of Bloomsbury Publishing Plc

Copyright © Dr Amit Bhushan Sharma and Ambika Rikhye, 2025
Foreword copyright © Boman Irani, 2025

Dr Amit Bhushan Sharma and Ambika Rikhye have asserted their moral rights to be identified
as the authors of this work in accordance with the Indian Copyright Act, 1957.

Some names and details of individuals have been changed to preserve their anonymity.

All rights reserved. No part of this publication may be: i) reproduced or transmitted in any
form, electronic or mechanical, including photocopying, recording or by means of any
information storage or retrieval system without prior permission in writing from the publishers;
or ii) used or reproduced in any way for the training, development or operation of artificial
intelligence (AI) technologies, including generative AI technologies. The rights holders
expressly reserve this publication from the text and data mining exception as per Article 4(3) of
the Digital Single Market Directive (EU) 2019/790

Bloomsbury Publishing Plc does not have any control over, or responsibility for, any third-
party websites referred to in this book. All internet addresses given in this book were correct at
the time of going to press. The author and publisher regret any inconvenience caused if
addresses have changed or sites have ceased to exist, but can accept no responsibility for any
such changes.

This book is intended for informational and educational purposes only. It does not provide
personalised medical advice, diagnosis or treatment. The content within this book should not be
considered a substitute for professional medical advice, diagnosis or treatment.

Always seek the advice of your physician or other qualified health provider with any questions
you may have regarding a medical condition. Never disregard professional medical advice or
delay in seeking it because of something you have read in this book.

The author and publisher do not assume any liability for any injury, illness or damage incurred
directly or indirectly from the use or application of the information contained in this book. It is
recommended to consult with a qualified healthcare professional before implementing any
suggestions or recommendations presented in this book.

ISBN: PB: 978-93-69522-27-9; ebook: 978-93-69528-39-4

2 4 6 8 10 9 7 5 3 1

Typeset in Bembo Std Manipal Technologies Limited
Printed and bound in India by Gopsons Papers Pvt. Ltd., Noida

To find out more about our authors and books visit www.bloomsbury.com and
sign up for our newsletters

When you lock eyes with the one you adore,
Your heart flutters wildly, craving them more.

When you share that first kiss, soft and sweet,
Your heart skips a beat, a moment complete.

When you hear your baby's heartbeat, steady and strong,
Your heart overflows, a love lifelong.

When your baby cries for the very first time,
Your heart melts gently, pure and sublime.

When a loved one falls ill, the fear runs deep,
Your heart feels heavy, the pain won't sleep.

When you feel close and the secrets pour out,
Your heart starts trusting, leaving no doubt.

And when a loved one is no longer near,
Your heart aches softly, cherishing them dear.

Ambika Rikhye

Contents

Message from J.P. Nadda — ix
Foreword by Boman Irani — xi
Why We Decided to Write This Book — xiii

PART ONE MATTERS OF THE HEART: REAL STORIES, REAL LESSONS

1. Ticking Time Bomb: How One Man's Denial Cost Him Everything — 3
2. A Race Against Time: Sandhya's Battle for Every Breath — 8
3. Defying the Unthinkable: Power Athlete Dhriti's Hidden Battle — 13
4. Shattered Rhythm: The Unseen Battle Behind the Mic — 16
5. Too Young to Fall: The Catastrophic Heartbreak — 21
6. The Poisoned Cure — 24
7. Like Father, Like Son: A Fight Against Recurrence — 27
8. The Fallen Star: Heartbreak on the Field — 30
9. Pregnancy and the Heart — 36
10. Beyond the Reps: Gym and Sudden Cardiac Deaths — 42
11. Miracle at the Airport: When Time Was Running Out — 47
12. Unpacking Obesity: The Struggles, Science and Sustainable Solutions — 51
13. Stress Testing Your Heart: A Vital Step for Busy Executives — 57
14. From Health to Hospital: A Fit Life Takes a Sudden Twist — 64
15. Heart Attack After Surgery — 67
16. Blue Babies and an Asymptomatic Adult — 73
17. When Emotions Hurt the Heart: Understanding Broken Heart Syndrome — 82

18.	Beyond Snoring: A Scary Wake-Up Call	87
19.	Women and Heart Attacks	94
20.	Right Heart Failure in Alcoholic Liver Disease	102
21.	A Pregnancy Complicated by Rheumatic Heart Disease	111
22.	A Second Chance: Treating Heart Failure and Severe Mitral Regurgitation with MitraClip	117
23.	Life 2.0: How a Seventy-Six-Year-Old Beat Heart Trouble with a Simple Procedure	123

PART TWO SCIENCE OF THE HEART: LIVING STRONGER, LIVING LONGER

24.	Sleep and the Heart	131
25.	Exercise and the Heart	136
26.	Pollution and the Heart	143
27.	Food and Heart Health	148
28.	Hearty Recipes	153
29.	Can Heart Diseases Be Reversed?	164
30.	Sudden Deaths in Young People	168
31.	Palpitations	174
32.	Breathing and Meditation	180
33.	Heart Health in Perimenopause and Menopause	186
34.	Varicose Veins	193
35.	Valvular Heart Disease	202
36.	Mending the Holes in the Heart: Device Closure Versus Surgery	211
37.	Chest Pain	218
38.	Coronary Artery Bypass Surgery	225
39.	Understanding Pericardial Effusion	231
40.	When Your Heart Skips a Beat – And Not in a Romantic Way	238
41.	Decoding Coronary Angiography: Why It Matters	243

Notes	249
About the Authors	255

Message from J.P. Nadda, Minister of Health and Family Welfare

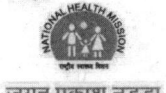

जगत प्रकाश नड्डा
JAGAT PRAKASH NADDA

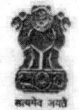

मंत्री
स्वास्थ्य एवं परिवार कल्याण
व रसायन एवं उर्वरक
भारत सरकार
Minister
Health & Family Welfare
and Chemicals & Fertilizers
Government of India

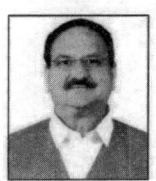

MESSAGE

I am happy to note that Dr. Amit Bhushan Sharma, one of the respected Cardiologist of the country, has authored book – "Heartbeat". With over 25 years of distinguished practice, Dr. Amit Bhushan Sharma has been at the forefront of structural heart and complex coronary interventions, saving countless lives and shaping the future of cardiovascular care.

This book is not just a reflection of his vast clinical expertise, but also his deep commitment to public health and patient education. By distilling complex medical knowledge into practical guidance, Dr. Amit Bhushan Sharma empowers readers to take charge of their heart health and live healthier lives.

(Jagat Prakash Nadda)

Foreword

A FLUTTER. A SKIP. A THUD.
We've all felt our hearts speak a language of their own – whether it's the excitement of love, the terror of loss or the weight of waiting for a doctor to walk in with news that might change everything.

What this book does so beautifully is that it doesn't drown you in jargon or overwhelm you with fear.

Instead, it tells stories – real, raw and unforgettable. It takes you from the sterile corridors of hospitals into the inner chambers of the human spirit.

You'll meet people who ignored warning signs, those who fought back against impossible odds and those whose lives were saved because someone performed CPR at the right time. And then, just when you think it is all about disease, the book gently shifts gears and shows you the road map to prevention, clarity and control – through sleep, food, stress management and lifestyle changes.

It is not just for patients. It is for all of us who have ignored a racing heart, blamed palpitations on anxiety or postponed a check-up 'until next month'.

What I love most is how *Heartbeat* never forgets that behind every diagnosis is a daughter, a friend, a father, a lover – a human. That in the end the heart is not just an organ. It is the seat of our emotions, our stories and, sometimes, our second chances.

This book has the power to save lives – not just through its medical insight but also through its compassion.

This book listens to your heartbeat – and tells you how to keep it strong.

Boman Irani
Award-winning actor, producer, director and screenwriter

Why We Decided to Write This Book

Dr Amit Bhushan Sharma

Heart disease is often thought of as a problem for older adults or those with obvious risk factors like diabetes or obesity. However, in my years as a cardiologist, I have seen heart conditions affect people of all ages and backgrounds – sometimes in the most unexpected ways. I have met young athletes who suffered heart attacks, fit individuals who ignored early symptoms and children whose heart defects went undiagnosed until it was too late.

This book is for everyone – not just patients or doctors but also parents, carers and anyone who wants to understand their heart better. The human heart beats more than 100,000 times a day, yet most of us only think about it when something goes wrong. The purpose of this book is simple: to explain heart health in a way that is clear, practical and free of medical jargon so that people can make informed decisions about their well-being.

This book is dedicated to the patients who never had the chance to get better:

To the young lives lost without warning,

To the elderly who mistook their breathlessness for asthma,

And to the women whose 'acidity' masked silent, fatal heart disease.

They were the anomalies – undiagnosed, unheard – simply because they lacked access to the right information or the time to act.

In cardiology, we say: Time is muscle. And knowledge? It can mean the difference between life and death.

With this book, I hope to educate, to empower, and to offer readers a better chance – to recognise the signs, to act swiftly, and perhaps, to save a life.

I also extend my deepest gratitude to my family –

To my parents, Dr Dharam Bhushan Sharma and Dr Kumkum Sharma,

To my wife, Dr Shalini Sharma,

And to my daughters, Pranaya, Prisha and Palmira –

For being my unwavering source of strength, inspiration and love through every step of this journey.

This work is as much yours as it is mine.

Ambika Rikhye

We often wander through life with a sense of 'having it all', taking the simplest pleasures for granted. We indulge in candy and sweets, savouring the sugary delight until the harsh realities of cavities and tooth decay ruin our pleasure. We get lost in a sea of screens – scrolling, binge-watching and distracting ourselves – until our fatigued eyes give up. In the rush and bustle of our daily routines, it is all too easy to overlook the long-term consequences of choices we make and forget that each moment is a gift to enjoy and protect.

Life felt wonderfully smooth as I lovingly shaped my child's little world – our days filled with joyful learning, cheering for green veggies and cosy story times that we both adored. I thought I had every day perfectly planned. Then, one morning, an unexpected event shattered my sense of control. I was told that my father had had a heart attack the previous night. When I found out he was in the intensive care unit (ICU), panic swept over me.

One of my greatest sources of strength had always been my father, a man who diligently controlled his hypertension and diabetes and went on daily walks. The fragility of his health, however, as I realised in that moment, was something I had unintentionally overlooked since I was so preoccupied with taking care of my child.

My heart was heavy with the hard reality. I sensed a persistent shadow of fear, even after my father miraculously recovered and returned home two days later. I needed some time to process the emotional turmoil the incident had caused, but it also made me realise how important it is to look after my needs in addition to those of my family.

Let us pause for a moment, individuals everywhere: maintaining our health is not an option; it is a need. We can only live a healthy and meaningful life when we take care of our bodies and minds. That is why I have chosen to partner with Dr Amit Bhushan Sharma on an issue that resonates deeply with me. Together, we hope to raise awareness that adopting a healthier lifestyle can prevent many issues from occurring and that heart health is a journey we can conquer.

Join us in this critical attempt as we unlock the secrets to a strong and fit heart to empower you and your loved ones to live life to the fullest. After all, healthy people are the foundation of a healthy family.

I would like to dedicate this book to my husband, Rohit. Now, I finally understand why you wake up at 5 AM to go for a run. As I write this dedication, sipping a glass of wine, you're still at the gym, working out. One of us is clearly taking cardiac health a lot more seriously.

A few words of appreciation for my family members – for teaching me that finding humour in everyday chaos is the ultimate food for the soul (and, of course, a happy heart)!

Let us embark on this journey together!

Disclaimer: Each story in this book is real and deeply personal. To protect the individuals who trusted us with their journeys, we've changed the names and any identifying details.

PART ONE

MATTERS OF THE HEART: REAL STORIES, REAL LESSONS

1

Ticking Time Bomb: How One Man's Denial Cost Him Everything

TIME IS MUSCLE IN 'heart attacks'. Every minute is critical. The longer the heart attack goes untreated, the more the heart muscle gets damaged. There are two key concepts in acute heart attack cases. One is door-to-needle time – the time interval between the patient's arrival at the hospital and the time the treatment is started. This should be less than 30 minutes.

The other key concept is 'door to balloon time', the time interval between the patient arriving at the hospital and the patient undergoing a procedure like an angioplasty (to open blocked arteries with a stent). It should ideally be less than 90 minutes.

There are five psychological stages that a patient usually experiences when they are dealing with a heart attack.

1. Denial: The patient refuses to believe that they have had a heart attack.
2. Anger: The patient questions why this is happening to them.
3. Bargaining: The patient is coming to terms with what has happened, but there is still a lot of inner conflict.
4. Depression: The patient feels sad or hopeless about their situation.
5. Acceptance: The patient finally accepts their situation and is ready to undergo treatment.

The sooner a patient transitions from denial to acceptance, the better the odds of successful therapy and recovery. Speedier acceptance leads to earlier medical action, which is critical for a successful outcome.

In the heart-stopping world of life-threatening medical emergencies, time is more than simply a concern; it is a constant foe. When a heart attack occurs, every second that passes without treatment is a blow to the heart's very being. Ravi Aggarwal's story is a stark testimonial to this harsh reality, in which a moment's delay almost lost him his life. His tragedy not only reveals the perilous junction of current health concerns but also emphasises the critical necessity for immediate action and acute awareness. We dig into the tragic path of a young man whose life was on the line and try to demonstrate the vital interplay of symptoms, medical intervention and often-overlooked risk factors.

The patient, Ravi Aggarwal, a thirty-six-year-old male, appeared with acute chest pain extending to his left arm, accompanied by uneasiness, sweating and a sense of impending doom (referred to as *ghabrahat* in Hindi).

He had experienced similar symptoms one or two days before admission and was told to seek emergency care since his electrocardiogram (ECG, a simple test where small sensors are placed on your skin to record the heart's electrical activity) revealed signs of a heart attack, but he ignored the symptoms because he needed to be there for his son's dental appointment.

The narrative that follows sheds light on the crucial role diabetes plays in the health issues that younger populations experience as well as the importance of recognising early symptoms.

Case Overview: Ravi Aggarwal's Close Call

Ravi's initial diagnosis revealed significant cardiovascular issues, including double vessel disease (there are three blood vessels, two on the left supplying about 80 per cent to the heart and one on the right supplying about 20 per cent). The patient's cardiac function was normal when he had come the night before, but overnight, he got heart failure with a reduced heart function (HFrEF) of 32 per cent (normal functionality should be 60 per cent). His medical history includes type 2 diabetes, which is an established risk factor for cardiovascular disease. Immediate procedures, including coronary angiography (a procedure that allows doctors to see the blood vessels of the heart) and coronary angioplasty (percutaneous transluminal coronary angioplasty) with stent implantation, were completed successfully.

The Silent Killer: How Hidden Dangers Escalated the Crisis

Diabetes is an important factor that increases the risk of heart disease. High blood sugar levels can damage blood vessels and nerves that control the heart, resulting in disorders including atherosclerosis (a build-up of fatty deposits, cholesterol and other substances within the walls of arteries, causing them to narrow and stiffen). Ravi's glycated haemoglobin (HbA1c) level was significantly raised at 11 per cent, indicating poor blood sugar control in the previous months. This chronic hyperglycaemia likely contributed to the rapid progression of his cardiovascular disease.

When the Body's Alarms Go Unheard

The symptoms experienced by Ravi, such as left-sided chest pain radiating to the arm, uneasiness and sweating, are classic indicators of a heart attack. To avoid serious consequences, these symptoms must be promptly identified and treated. Sadly, a lot of young adults choose to ignore these warning signs, thinking that the causes are likely not as serious because they are younger.

On the Brink: Battling His Way Back from the Edge

During his hospital stay, Ravi received dual antiplatelet therapy, statins and other supportive treatments. In general, angiography is like passing a hot knife through butter, but in patients with diabetes, the vessel is so heavily calcified that the guide wire has difficulty passing through. Following the intervention, Ravi's condition stabilised, and he was released with a detailed pharmaceutical plan to control his diabetes and cardiac disease. However, he later presented with an acute onset of weakness on the left side of his body and slurred speech, indicating a stroke, which necessitated further treatment, including thrombolysis.

The Hidden Dangers to the Heart Threatening a Generation

Ravi Aggarwal's case reflects the concerning trend of a rise in cardiovascular incidents among adults with diabetes. It emphasises the importance of diabetes awareness and proactive management of cardiovascular risk factors in this population. Regular blood glucose monitoring, a balanced diet and regular physical activity are all important preventative measures. Furthermore, recognising and responding quickly to the symptoms of a heart attack can dramatically improve results.

The Learning

The link between diabetes and cardiovascular disease in young adults is a major threat to public health. Healthcare professionals must emphasise the importance of lifestyle changes and following medical advice to reduce the risks of diabetes and heart disease. By doing so, we aim to decrease the frequency of such life-threatening events in the younger population.

Vital Life-Saving Lessons for Everyone

1. Diabetic patients will not always experience typical symptoms. They may get a heart attack without the usual warning signs.

2. Fasting blood sugar, blood pressure and pulse must be monitored at home.
3. The prevalence of heart attacks in young individuals with comorbidities has shifted paradigms.
4. 'Time is muscle.' If the patient had come for assistance at the initial onset of symptoms, there would have been less damage. The delay in treatment further contributes to an elevated risk of stroke (as happened in this case).
5. There is no medication that can improve the heart's pumping function.

Heart attacks are no longer limited to older people, as Ravi's terrifying experience with heart disease reminds us. This account of a potentially fatal catastrophe brings to light a sad reality: even those who appear unbreakable can be susceptible. Evidently, prompt medical attention, mindfulness about your body's warning signs and early detection are not just options – they are necessities. His tale serves as a strong reminder to all of us to pay attention to the warning indications and take prompt action. Accepting these teachings can mean the difference between life and death in a world where every heartbeat matters.

> 'Did you know that the 7,570.82 litres of blood that your heart pumps every day travels about 19,312 kilometres through your body each day?'[1]
>
> Cleveland Clinic[1]

2

A Race Against Time: Sandhya's Battle for Every Breath

WHEN SANDHYA DHRUVE ENTERED the hospital, she had no idea that her body was a battleground concealing a dark secret. What started off as a little pain quickly turned into a scary experience. Her pulse was beating faster as if alerting her to something much more hazardous than what was visible, and a feeling of dread was creeping in with every shallow breath. She had no idea that she was poised on the brink of something terrible and silent waiting to strike. Her physicians recognised the urgency, but the battle for her life was just getting started, and the full extent of the situation would not become clear for some time.

Case Overview

Sandhya Dhruve, a thirty-five-year-old professional and mother, arrived at the hospital with disturbing symptoms of breathlessness, discomfort and palpitations that had lasted three to four days. What appeared to be minor symptoms quickly escalated, indicating a considerably more dangerous underlying medical condition.

Sandhya's pulmonary angiography revealed a serious near-total obstruction of the right pulmonary artery, indicating a severe and potentially fatal blockage. The discovery of segmental thrombosis (clots) complicated her condition, demanding immediate attention. To quickly restore normal blood flow to her lungs, a mechanical thrombectomy was performed, successfully removing the clots and lowering the risk of future problems.

The Deadly Spiral of Pulmonary Embolism

1. Severity of blockage: In Sandhya's case, the near-complete obstruction of the right pulmonary artery is one of the most serious types of pulmonary embolism, in which a clot got dislodged from her leg and travelled to her lungs. This kind of obstruction can quickly lead to life-threatening consequences, such as right-sided heart failure, as the heart tries to cope with the increased pressure and demand.
2. Contributing risk factors: Sandhya was taking oral contraceptive pills to treat adenomyosis (a gynaecological condition in which the uterine lining grows into the muscle of the uterine wall), and these pills are a known risk factor for thrombosis. They raise the risk of blood clot formation, particularly in women with other risk factors such as smoking, obesity or a history of thromboembolic events.
3. Symptom manifestation: Sandhya's sudden onset of breathing difficulties and palpitations are classic hallmarks of pulmonary embolism, but the severity of her condition raised immediate concern. These symptoms, which are frequently indicative of a significant underlying condition, should never be ignored and demand immediate medical attention.
4. Advanced diagnostic imaging: The pulmonary angiography, which is the gold standard for diagnosing pulmonary embolism, showed clear and comprehensive images of the lung's blood vessels. Sandhya's angiography revealed a near-complete blockage, emphasising the importance of urgent surgical intervention.

The Surgical Strike: Mechanical Thrombectomy's Critical Role

Mechanical thrombectomy is a cutting-edge, minimally invasive surgery that involves inserting a catheter into a blood vessel and physically extracting the clot. This method is critical in severe or high-risk cases of pulmonary embolism, especially when thrombolytic treatment is unsuccessful or not recommended. The surgery saved Sandhya's life by successfully restoring blood flow and considerably reducing the chance of future problems.

Deep Vein Thrombosis: The Hidden Assassin

In addition to her pulmonary embolism, Sandhya's lower limb Doppler ultrasound revealed deep vein thrombosis, which is often the precursor to pulmonary embolism. Deep vein thrombosis occurs when a blood clot forms in the deep veins, typically in the legs. If left untreated, parts of the clot can break off and travel to the lungs, causing a pulmonary embolism.

Deep Vein Thrombosis: Crucial Takeaways

1. The hidden triggers: Deep vein thrombosis is frequently associated with extended immobility, the use of certain drugs such as oral contraceptives, recent surgery and hereditary predisposition.
2. Warning signs: This condition can cause swelling, discomfort, redness and warmth in the affected limb, but it can also remain asymptomatic, making it silent but serious.
3. Decoding the silent killer: Doppler ultrasonography is the standard diagnostic tool for diagnosing deep vein thrombosis. Anticoagulant medication is commonly used to prevent additional clot formation and lower the risk of pulmonary embolism.

On the Frontlines: Defeating the Threat Through Awareness and Prevention

Sandhya's example reminds us how important it is to recognise the warning signs and symptoms of both pulmonary embolism and deep vein thrombosis. It emphasises the necessity of raising awareness of the risk factors for these illnesses. Women, particularly those who use oral contraceptives, must recognise the possible risks and remain vigilant in checking for early symptoms.

Preventative Measures

1. Lifestyle changes: Regular physical activity, maintenance of a healthy weight and avoidance of prolonged periods of immobility can significantly reduce the risk of deep vein thrombosis and subsequent pulmonary embolism.
2. Medical supervision: Regular check-ups and consultations with healthcare professionals are critical for managing and decreasing associated risks, particularly for people taking medications such as oral contraceptives.
3. Raise public awareness: Educational campaigns focusing on the signs, symptoms and risk factors of deep vein thrombosis and pulmonary embolism can encourage earlier detection and intervention, thus saving countless lives.

The Endgame: The Fight for Life and the Power of Early Intervention

Sandhya Dhruve's battle with pulmonary embolism and deep vein thrombosis serves as a powerful reminder of the critical importance that early discovery, prompt medical intervention and ongoing awareness play in saving lives. Her story emphasises the significance of being vigilant in recognising symptoms and identifying the risk factors. As Sandhya recovers, her tale will undoubtedly raise awareness and contribute to better outcomes for others facing similar health risks.

Although Sandhya fell into danger quickly, her stunning recovery from the edge was nearly unthinkable. This was no longer a terrifying unknown; it was a war fought with skill, speed and unwavering determination that could mean the difference between life and death. Her medical intervention saved her from what had appeared like an imminent disaster as all the components of her disease came together. Life is fragile, and danger may be concealed in plain sight and strike without notice. Alertness and quick decision-making can be the only things separating survival from a far more sinister end.

> 'Arteries are only about 4 millimeters in diameter. It doesn't take too much of those fatty, greasy foods over the period to start clogging up the arteries.'
> Roger Blumenthal, MD (Johns Hopkins cardiologist)[1]

3

Defying the Unthinkable: Power Athlete Dhriti's Hidden Battle

DHRITI, A FORTY-SEVEN-YEAR-OLD woman whose name means 'unmatched strength and determination', has long been recognised for her extraordinary achievements. Her resumé showed her continuous dedication: she trekked to the Everest Base Camp, finished the arduous Ironman triathlon in Vietnam and completed five swimathons in the challenging waters of Goa.

She exercised, cycled and walked tirelessly for days on end, each step reflecting her steadfast commitment to success and well-being. Dhriti represented athletic strength to the entire world and was a live example of the phrase 'mind over matter'.

The Silent Storm

Yet, behind the facade of physical prowess lay a storm that threatened to shatter her world. Dhriti had battled resistant hypertension for years, a condition that seemed to defeat the effects of even the strongest antihypertensive drugs. Her blood pressure persisted as a ruthless enemy despite her following doctors' strict instructions and routinely taking more than three drugs. This was a serious personal dilemma rather than just a health problem. It seemed cruelly ironic to her that she would have to live with a condition overriding her freedom to do as she pleased.

Resistant hypertension is more than just a medical diagnosis; it is a warning sign of an approaching disaster. It brings up the dangers of kidney illness, heart attacks and strokes – threats that loomed large over Dhriti's athletic endeavours like dark clouds. Every spike in blood pressure felt like a ticking time bomb, an alarming signal that any physical accomplishments she may make could easily be eclipsed by an invisible enemy.

A Ray of Hope: The Search for Cutting-Edge Care

The usual treatments looked increasingly ineffective as her illness worsened. Her medical team was presented with an extremely difficult task: figuring out a way to give hope in the face of conventional procedures failing. At that point, they put out a groundbreaking strategy: renal denervation therapy.

A newly introduced minimally invasive technique called renal denervation aims at restructuring the nerves in the renal arteries, which are vital for controlling blood pressure. Patients like Dhriti, who run out of choices, can find a lifeline with this surgery. This was not only a medical treatment but also a chance to regain her health and resume her athletic adventure free from the weight of hypertension.

A Story of Determination: Dhriti's Unbreakable Spirit

Dhriti's story goes beyond medical accomplishments and exemplifies the resilience of the human spirit. Her unwavering determination to conquer resistant hypertension serves as an important reminder that even the most difficult obstacles can be overcome. Her swimathons, marathons and epic climbs are not just achievements but turning points in a remarkable journey of determination.

Dhriti continues to move against the tide and live life on her own terms. Her spirit is unaffected by the difficulties she has faced, and she is still as adventurous and active as ever. This narrative is very inspiring and illustrates both the effectiveness of cutting-edge medical treatments and the strength of the human spirit. Even in the face of overwhelming difficulty, great triumphs can be achieved through hope, hard work and the right support.

Dhriti's entire life, from the summit of Everest to the depths of personal hardships, reaffirms that success is always attainable with bravery and correct support.

> 'Hypertension is a major cause of premature death worldwide. Hypertension is diagnosed if, when it is measured on two different days, the systolic blood pressure readings on both days is ≥140 mmHg and/or the diastolic blood pressure readings on both days is ≥90 mmHg.'
> World Health Organisation[1]

4

Shattered Rhythm: The Unseen Battle Behind the Mic

ARAVI MEHTA WAS a driven eighteen-year-old college student who had a passion for public speaking. She was well known for her charm and eloquence, and at her institution, she was frequently chosen to host events and debates. However, every event was accompanied by a crippling feeling of anxiety. She would find it difficult to breathe due to the intense pounding of her heart. Everyone, including Aravi, explained it away as stage fright, a normal case of anxiety before taking centre stage.

Heart in Crisis: The Hidden Turmoil Behind Stage Fright

Aravi's 'stage fright' was different, though. It went beyond nervousness before a speech. Intense palpitations occasionally left her feeling as though her heart was pounding uncontrollably, even off stage. She endured it anyway, thinking it to be the pressure of giving a performance in front of large audiences.

During a campus debate one day, Aravi's heart started racing more quickly than it had ever done. Her vision became blurred, and she started to feel dizzy. She quickly excused herself and hurried to the restrooms, where she splashed cold water on her face, hoping that it would soothe her. However, it didn't. Her heart continued to race, and soon she was having trouble breathing. A friend saw her in distress just in time and took her to the campus clinic.

The Awakening: Discovering the True Nature of Anxiety

When the nurse at the clinic took her pulse, it was dangerously high – more than 200 beats per minute. As she realised how serious it was, she called for an ambulance to take Aravi to the hospital. Following a battery of tests, doctors at the hospital concluded that Aravi had supraventricular tachycardia, a condition in which the heart beats abnormally rapidly due to abnormal electrical pathways.

Finding Clarity: The Diagnosis That Redefined Fear

Aravi was taken aback. She was unaware that what she had believed to be stage fright or anxiety for a long time was a cardiac condition. The doctors clarified that although anxiety can worsen the symptoms, an electrical short circuit in her heart was the actual cause. They recommended an extended loop recorder to track her heart's electrical activity over a few days to confirm the diagnosis and establish the optimal course of treatment.

Even during Aravi's periods of relaxation, the extended loop recorder showed recurrent episodes of supraventricular tachycardia. The doctors suggested an ablation treatment, in which catheters would be used to cut off the aberrant electrical pathways causing irregular heartbeats. Aravi was terrified about having heart surgery, but she knew she had to stop living in constant fear of another incident.

The Day Everything Changed

The day of the procedure came, and with the support of her family and friends, Aravi underwent the ablation. Aravi noticed a difference practically immediately after the successful operation. She appeared to be free of the ongoing anxiousness that had been plaguing her for years. She could now stand in front of people without fearing that her heart might turn against her.

Aravi discovered 'vagal manoeuvres' in the weeks that followed her recovery. These methods, which include bearing down (trying to breathe out with your stomach muscles but not allowing air out of your nose or mouth), sprinkling cold water on the face and holding breath, can help stop a supraventricular tachycardia attack by stimulating the vagus nerve. While these manoeuvres are beneficial in managing abrupt episodes, they are temporary fixes, and Aravi realised that the ablation was the true remedy for her illness.

From Patient to Advocate: Aravi's New Mission in Life

Aravi got her heart back in beat and faced life with new-found self-assurance. She not only recovered but also developed a new passion for educating people about cardiac problems that affect young people. She began a blog where she discussed her experience and gave people advice on how to tell the difference between anxiety and underlying medical concerns.

Today, Aravi is a successful TV anchor, known for her calm demeanour and sharp interviewing skills. Her transformation from a college student who struggled with stage fright to a self-assured television personality is remarkable. She frequently shares her story of supraventricular tachycardia, urging people to pay attention to their bodies and get help if something feels wrong.

From Darkness to Dawn: Aravi's Path of Courage and Lasting Impact

Aravi's story is a powerful reminder that not all health issues are what they seem. While anxiety is genuine and can be extremely crippling, occasionally, its symptoms can indicate something more serious. For Aravi, knowing that changed everything, transforming what may have been a tale of struggle into one of victory and hope.

To ensure a clear understanding of the terms mentioned in this chapter, we have included these definitions for quick reference and deeper understanding.

Palpitations

Palpitations refer to the sensation of feeling your own heartbeat and can be described as a rapid, irregular or forceful heartbeat. Some people may feel like their heart is fluttering, pounding or skipping beats. Palpitations can occur due to various reasons, ranging from benign to more serious underlying conditions.

Causes of Palpitations

Cardiac Causes

1. Arrhythmias (for example, supraventricular tachycardia, ventricular tachycardia, atrial fibrillation [AFib])
2. Heart disease (for example, coronary artery disease [CAD], heart failure)
3. Valvular heart disease
4. Cardiomyopathy

Non-Cardiac Causes

1. Stress, anxiety or panic attacks
2. Excessive caffeine or alcohol consumption
3. Stimulant medications or recreational drugs
4. Hormonal changes (for example, during pregnancy, menopause or thyroid disorders)
5. Fever, dehydration or electrolyte imbalances
6. Anaemia

Supraventricular Tachycardia

This is a form of irregular heartbeat, also known as an arrhythmia, in which the heart's upper chambers (atria) beat unusually fast, frequently between 150 and 250 beats per minute.

Symptoms

These can include palpitations, dizziness, shortness of breath, chest discomfort or even fainting in severe cases.

Is it lethal?

The condition is usually not life-threatening but can be uncomfortable and alarming. It can sometimes require treatment to prevent recurrent episodes.

Ventricular Tachycardia

It is a rapid heart rate that originates in the ventricles (the lower chambers of the heart). The heart rate is often over 100 beats per minute with potentially dangerous consequences.

Symptoms

Symptoms are similar to supraventricular tachycardia but can be more severe, including chest pain, shortness of breath, dizziness and loss of consciousness.

Is it lethal?

Yes, it can be life-threatening, especially if it leads to ventricular fibrillation, which can cause sudden cardiac arrest if not treated immediately.

> 'It is my view and my personal clinical experience that anxiety disorders can play a major role in heart disease.'
> Una D. McCann, MD
> (Johns Hopkins Bayview Medical Centre)[1]

5

Too Young to Fall: The Catastrophic Heartbreak

The Nightmare Before Dawn

The clock struck 9 PM, signalling the end of a long day. The squad was winding down, tired but satisfied after hours of hard labour. The tranquillity was abruptly broken by the urgent clamour outside. The commotion signalled the entrance of a young man – barely twenty-five years old. He was rushed in from the emergency room (ER) – lifeless, without a pulse and with no measurable blood pressure. The air was tense as relentless cardiopulmonary resuscitation (CPR) continued.

The diagnosis? A massive myocardial infarction (heart attack). It seemed almost unbelievable – Ravi Malhotra, a young, married man with no apparent risk factors, now clinging to the edge of life.

The team had one option: fight with everything they had.

Time was running out. So it was decided to send Ravi into the catheterisation lab, where he would get constant CPR compressions and artificial supports.

One hour later, a miracle began to unfold. The team managed to open his artery, which had been 100 per cent blocked. Slowly, his blood pressure returned. The night itself held its breath, and the ventilator was removed the next morning. Ravi opened his eyes. He was alive.

Relief washed over the team, but a question loomed: Why did this happen to someone so young?

Unveiling the Mystery: No Risk Factors, Only Questions

This wasn't the typical case. The patient had:
1. no high blood pressure,
2. no diabetes,
3. no smoking history and
4. no family history of heart disease.

Ravi was, by all accounts, the picture of health. Then came a clue – a conversation with his father. The story revealed the hidden secret. The man's wife had left him, and they were on the verge of divorce. Their four-month-old daughter was caught in the crossfire of a crumbling relationship. Could a *broken heart* be the reason for this?

A Meeting That Changed Everything

I requested to speak to Ravi's wife. Hesitant but relenting, she agreed to come. I made a heartfelt plea: 'For the next few months, whatever happens between you two, please stay by his side. Hold his hand. Be there.'

Reluctantly, the couple began meeting in the outpatient department. Gradually, they started understanding each other. Minor adjustments, open conversations and shared experiences began to mend the cracks. Over time, they rediscovered their bond.

Now, four years later, their daughter is a happy four-and-a-half-year-old, and the couple is still together, stronger than ever.

The Ghosts Within: A Genetic Reveal

Determined to find the underlying cause, the medical team conducted advanced genetic testing. The results were startling. Ravi's chromosomes were severely damaged. His genetic age was seventy plus, though his physical age was just twenty-five. The culprit was a defective enzyme called *telomerase*, responsible for maintaining chromosomal integrity.

But why had telomerase failed? The answer lay not in his body but in his mind. Psychosocial stress, loneliness and the deprivation of love had wreaked havoc at a cellular level, ageing him decades beyond his years.

Loneliness: The Hidden Pandemic

This case highlights a critical truth: *loneliness* is the biggest pandemic of our times. Chronic stress and emotional turmoil can damage the heart as much as – or even more than – traditional risk factors. Cortisol, the body's stress hormone, fuels inflammation, endothelial dysfunction and plaque formation, leading to heart attacks in even the youngest of individuals.

Lessons from the Heart

This story isn't just about saving a life; it is about saving a family. It is about how love, support and connection can heal wounds that medicine alone cannot. It serves as a reminder that emotional well-being is as crucial as physical health. Young individuals are not immune to heart disease. Loneliness, heartbreak and unresolved stress can literally break the heart. As the couple's journey reminds us, healing often begins with holding hands and letting go of hurt.

Final Thought: A Call to Action

We must place a higher priority on connection in a world that is becoming more and more divided by screens, lonely because of hectic lives and tense due to unfulfilled expectations. Loneliness is a silent murderer in addition to being an emotional vacuum. Let us fight it, together.

> 'The beating sound from your heart – lub–dub, lub–dub, lub–dub – is from the clap of valve leaflets opening and closing.'[1]
>
> Cleveland Clinic[1]

6

The Poisoned Cure

A Sudden Call for Help

It was a quiet evening at home, the kind where nothing out of the ordinary was expected. The clock struck 10 PM, and I was at the dinner table when my phone buzzed insistently. On the other end was a close friend, his voice trembling and broken. A successful entrepreneur running multiple polyclinics, he was now in desperate need of help.

He had been at a restaurant with friends, enjoying drinks and snacks, when a sharp pain gripped his chest. Sweating profusely and barely able to breathe, he managed to reach the emergency room. His blood pressure was dangerously high at 180/90, and he couldn't sit still or lie down. His agony was written all over his face as he winced and writhed, unable to find relief.

The ECG didn't indicate a massive heart attack, yet something was seriously wrong. Medicines failed to ease his pain, leaving us no choice. By midnight, we prepared for an emergency angiogram. But where was his wife?

The Missing Wife

At 10:30 PM, I had called her. 'Your husband is in the emergency room. It is serious. Please come immediately,' I urged. She acknowledged the call but did not appear.

By 12:30 AM, our patience wore thin. His friend, who had been with him at dinner, gave consent for the procedure in her absence.

The angiogram revealed no major blockages – a moment of relief in the chaos. Still, he was shifted to the ICU for observation, his condition monitored closely. But there was no sign of his wife. Repeated calls went unanswered. When she finally answered, she replied casually, 'I'll come in the morning.'

The Morning After

At 10 AM the next day, she finally arrived. To my surprise, she walked into the ICU looking relaxed, her appearance polished and calm, as though nothing had happened. 'Everything is fine, right?' she asked, flashing a composed smile.

Her demeanour was so unexpected that I couldn't help but ask, 'Why didn't you come last night? Your husband was in immense pain, and we needed you.'

She paused for a moment, looked at me with an unwavering expression and dropped a bombshell that left me stunned.

The Wife's Secret Weapon

'I knew this day would come,' she said with chilling calmness. 'I was tired of his drinking habits, and he never listened to me, no matter how much I pleaded. So I decided to act. I mixed a drug called disulfiram into the flour he eats daily. It reacts violently with alcohol, causing the kind of symptoms you saw last night. I wanted to scare him into giving up drinking for good.'

I was speechless. She continued, 'I stayed home because I knew he wasn't having a heart attack. This was his lesson. And it seems to have worked, hasn't it?'

A Bold Gamble or a Reckless Act?

Even after a year, her husband had not touched a drop of alcohol. However, her method left me quite shaken. On the one hand, she had forced him to confront his dangerous habit. On the other hand, she had risked his health – and perhaps his life – to make her point.

The Debate

1. Caring or reckless? Was her act an extreme form of tough love, born out of frustration and desperation to save her husband from alcohol?
2. Dangerous or justified? Disulfiram reactions can mimic severe cardiac events, causing panic and unnecessary medical interventions. What if something had gone wrong during the episode?

A Lesson in Love and Limits

This story raises difficult questions about the lengths we go to for the people we care about. The wife's unconventional approach succeeded in stopping her husband's harmful habit, but it also sparks a debate about the methods she used and their implications.

Was It Love? Was It Determination? Or Was It Both?

In the end, perhaps it is a story not about right or wrong but about the grey areas we navigate in relationships, where emotions and intentions collide in unpredictable ways.

One thing is certain: This was a cure he'll *never* forget.

'Alcoholism affects people beyond just the person drinking. Friends, family and other people that a person suffering the effects of alcoholism interacts with on a regular basis are all likely to experience problems related to the condition.'

alcohol.org[1]

7

Like Father, Like Son: A Fight Against Recurrence

YOU WOULDN'T EXPECT A twenty-nine-year-old software developer like Raghav to be concerned about heart disease. Despite his struggles with weight and a sedentary lifestyle, he always believed he had time to 'get healthy' eventually because he was young and had his entire life ahead of him. But one terrible day forever changed his perspective on life.

One evening, Raghav's father experienced chest discomfort and required immediate hospitalisation. The diagnosis was a massive heart attack. Raghav and his family were traumatised by the incident, but fortunately, his father survived. Raghav decided to have a complete cardiovascular workup at the insistence of his father's physician. What he discovered shocked him.

A Shocking Discovery

The results were staggering. Raghav discovered he had alarmingly high levels of triglycerides, a critical red flag for heart disease, despite being in the prime of his life. Even more shocking was the revelation of elevated lipoprotein(a), or Lp(a), a genetic lipid particle akin to LDL (low-density lipoprotein) cholesterol but far more insidious, capable of igniting inflammation and clotting in arteries. Coupled with a cholesterol profile that alarmingly hinted at future danger, Raghav was faced with the harsh reality that he had inherited his family's troubling genetic legacy. He was at a heightened risk for premature cardiovascular events if he didn't take action.

The Fight for Survival

A high-intensity statin was prescribed by Raghav's doctor right away to lower his LDL cholesterol. The first line of treatment for cholesterol is statins, which function by preventing the liver from producing cholesterol. After taking statins for a few months, Raghav's triglycerides and Lp(a) levels remained stubbornly high, despite his hope that this would be sufficient on its own. His physician suggested inclisiran, a more recent drug made especially for patients like Raghav who are at high risk of cardiovascular problems even with regular treatment, based on his family history and blood tests.

Medication and New Hope

Inclisiran is a groundbreaking medication that reduces the PCSK9 (proprotein convertase subtilisin/kexin type 9) enzyme, which is important in the regulation of cholesterol, via a process known as siRNA (small interfering RNA). Inclisiran improves the activity of the liver's LDL receptors by lowering PCSK9 levels, which results in the removal of more LDL particles from the blood. For Raghav, this added weapon was vital because it not only helped to lower his LDL but also showed benefits in lowering his Lp(a) levels.

Medication was only one part of the therapeutic approach. Raghav's physician stressed the significance of altering his lifestyle. Raghav made a commitment to eating a healthier diet, avoiding sugar and processed foods, which were the main causes of his elevated triglycerides. In addition to working with a dietitian to emphasise heart-healthy meals high in fibre, omega-3 fatty acids and antioxidants, he established a regular exercise regimen, aiming for at least 150 minutes of moderate activity per week.

A Year of Change: Progress and Perseverance

Raghav's bloodwork improved significantly in just a year. Even his Lp(a) had decreased, and his triglyceride and LDL levels were under control. Although Raghav's father's heart attack scare served as a wake-up call, the path to these improvements wasn't simple. Five years later, he is a young man on a mission: not just to preserve his life but also to educate friends and family about genetic risks and heart disease prevention so they don't wait for a crisis to act. His body mass index (BMI) decreased to 23 from 29. He started out weighing 92 kg and now weighs 72 kg. Raghav's story serves as a reminder that although genetics play a significant role, proactive medical care and lifestyle modifications can have an enormous effect.

In the second part of this book, we uncover the essentials that shape a healthy life – exploring the power of food, the flow of exercise, the magic of sleep and so much more. Stay with us on this journey that transforms well-being into a way of life.

> 'Unlike pharmaceutical interventions that target specific pathways or risk factors, lifestyle modifications impact multiple risk factors simultaneously.'
> Ghodeshwar, Dube and Khobragade[1]

8

The Fallen Star: Heartbreak on the Field

ARYAN WAS A TALENTED young soccer player who was only nineteen years old. He was well known for his swiftness and endurance on the playing field. However, he abruptly collapsed during a fierce game, shocking his teammates and family. After being rushed to the hospital, Aryan was found to have hypertrophic cardiomyopathy (HCM), a medical condition that swells the heart muscle without causing any noticeable symptoms until it causes severe problems, including arrhythmias, fainting or even sudden cardiac arrest.

Since HCM is a genetic disorder, Aryan's treatment strategy focused heavily on his family history. According to doctors, the root cause is frequently genetic abnormalities that are passed down through families without any obvious symptoms until they appear out of nowhere. Aryan's heart collapsed as a result of outflow obstruction brought on by the stress of vigorous activity and his underlying medical condition.

The Significance of Genetic Screening

When Rohan, Aryan's older brother, found out about his sibling's illness, he became concerned. An athlete himself, he had never experienced symptoms, but Aryan's case made him realise that he, too, could be at risk. To check for HCM-related gene changes that may predispose people to similar occurrences, doctors advised Rohan and other family members to undergo genetic screening.

An essential first step in managing HCM in families is genetic screening. Finding these mutations can help determine who is at risk and guide medical care, monitoring and lifestyle changes. Even though Rohan had not yet displayed symptoms, genetic testing showed that he shared Aryan's mutation. Because of this early identification, Rohan's doctors were able to develop a proactive care plan that included frequent check-ups and recommended physical activity to reduce the likelihood of triggering symptoms.

Options for Treatment: Alcohol Ablation and Other Measures

Managing HCM was difficult for Aryan. He could take drugs to lessen his symptoms, but they wouldn't be sufficient to clear the blockage his thickening heart muscle was causing. Aryan was given two cutting-edge therapy choices by the doctors: alcohol septal ablation and surgical myectomy.

For some patients with obstructive HCM, alcohol septal ablation has emerged as a promising less invasive treatment option. This technique involves injecting a tiny quantity of alcohol into a specific septal artery, which causes the thickened heart muscle to contract and lessen blockage. According to Aryan's doctors, this alternative might help alleviate his discomfort and prevent significant surgery while improving his heart's blood flow. After careful consideration, Aryan decided on alcohol septal ablation.

Aryan saw a considerable improvement in his symptoms following the successful treatment. Even though he was unable to resume playing competitive soccer because of the possibility of further cardiac episodes, he was nevertheless able to have a more active and symptom-free life. His example also acted as a wake-up call for Rohan, who could better control his HCM risk with consistent monitoring and a specially designed fitness regimen.

Genetic Screening: A Life-saving Tool for Families

Aryan's story highlights the need for genetic screening and advanced treatment options like alcohol septal ablation in managing HCM. Many young athletes with HCM don't realise they have the problem until they have a major cardiac episode. Genetic screening may save lives by enabling at-risk family members to take preventative measures and get early interventions.

Today, Aryan and Rohan work together to raise awareness about HCM, urging other athletes and families to seek genetic testing when there's a family history of heart conditions. Aryan's story gives us a reminder of the impact that early identification and cutting-edge therapies can have on managing this complicated illness and lowering the likelihood of unexpected cardiac events in young, otherwise healthy people.

Hypertrophic Obstructive Cardiomyopathy (HOCM) in Young Athletes

HOCM is a heart condition that can have serious consequences, especially for young athletes. It is characterised by abnormal thickening of the heart muscle, primarily affecting the interventricular septum (the wall separating the left and right ventricles). This thickening in HOCM can block blood flow from the heart to the body, resulting in symptoms such as dizziness, exertion intolerance and blackouts. These symptoms are particularly dangerous for athletes who push themselves to the limit.

Understanding HOCM and How It Causes Symptoms

HOCM is a genetic condition, often inherited in an autosomal dominant pattern (people who are predisposed to this condition have a 50 per cent risk of passing it on to their offspring). Myocardial hypertrophy, or thicker heart muscle, is the result of this disease's abnormal genes causing the heart muscle cells to grow and become disorganised. The interventricular septum is usually more affected by the hypertrophy than the rest of the heart. Therefore, particularly during exercise or extreme exertion, the thicker septum may block blood flow out of the left ventricle (the heart's main pumping chamber).

This obstruction increases pressure in the left ventricle and causes turbulent blood flow, which can lead to the following symptoms:

1. Effort intolerance: The blockage causes blood flow to be reduced during exercise, which results in exhaustion, breathing difficulties and chest pain.
2. Syncope (blackouts): When the heart is exerted, it may not be able to pump enough blood, which can result in episodes of fainting.
3. Palpitations: Patients with HOCM may have arrhythmias, some of which may be fatal, as a result of abnormal electrical pathways in the thickened heart muscle.

Diagnosis of HOCM

For young athletes in particular, a precise diagnosis of HOCM is essential since, if left untreated, it can be fatal. The main diagnostic method is echocardiography, which shows thicker myocardium and may indicate the extent of blockage. Electrical abnormalities can be detected using ECG, and cardiac magnetic resonance imaging (MRI) may offer more precise imaging of the heart's anatomy. Exercise testing and 24-hour Holter monitoring can also be used to evaluate how the heart works when exercising.

Treatment of HOCM

The goals of HOCM treatment are to control risk, lessen symptoms and avoid sudden cardiac death. There are some important alternatives for treatment.

Medications

1. Beta-blockers (for example, metoprolol) are the first line of treatment and help reduce heart rate and left ventricular pressure, improving symptoms.
2. Calcium channel blockers (like verapamil) may also be used when beta-blockers are not enough, as they help relax the heart muscle.
3. Antiarrhythmics may be considered if there are significant arrhythmias, though caution is needed.

Septal Reduction Therapy

1. For patients with severe symptoms or high-risk HOCM that doesn't respond to medications, septal reduction procedures may be necessary.
2. Surgical myectomy involves removing part of the thickened septum to relieve obstruction, a procedure typically performed in specialised centres.
3. Alcohol septal ablation is a less invasive option where alcohol is injected into a small artery feeding the septum, causing part of the thickened muscle to shrink. This procedure can also relieve obstruction and improve blood flow.

Implantable Cardioverter-Defibrillator (ICD)

For those at high risk of sudden cardiac death due to arrhythmias, an ICD may be implanted. This device monitors the heart and can deliver shocks if life-threatening arrhythmias occur.

Lifestyle Modifications and Sports Restrictions

Athletes with HOCM often need to modify their activity levels. High-intensity sports are generally discouraged as the physical strain can increase the risk of arrhythmias and sudden cardiac death. Instead, moderate physical activity, focusing on non-competitive, low-impact exercises, may be allowed under medical guidance.

Risk of Sudden Cardiac Death

In young athletes, sudden cardiac death due to HOCM can occur, particularly during intense exertion. Recognising symptoms early and seeking evaluation can be life-saving. Genetic testing and family screening are also recommended as HOCM is often familial.

The Learning

HOCM is a complex and potentially dangerous condition, especially in young athletes. Awareness, early diagnosis and individualised treatment are essential to manage symptoms, reduce risks and help patients live safely. Proper medical care allows many young individuals with HOCM to enjoy active lives, albeit with certain lifestyle modifications to safeguard their health.

> 'When heart disease strikes Indians, it tends to do so at an earlier age (almost 33% earlier) than other demographics, often without prior warning. Furthermore, 50% of all heart attacks in Indian men occur under 50 years of age and 25% of all heart attacks in Indian men occur under 40 years of age, a staggering figure! Indian women have high mortality rates from cardiac disease as well.'
>
> Indian Heart Association[1]

9

Pregnancy and the Heart

A Mother's Unexpected Battle

Ananya, a thirty-two-year-old schoolteacher, had eagerly awaited the birth of her first child. Her pregnancy had been smooth, apart from mild fatigue and swelling in her legs, which her doctor assured her were normal. However, her journey took an unseen development after delivery.

Within a week of giving birth to a healthy baby boy, Ananya strangely struggled to catch her breath. At first, she dismissed it as exhaustion from sleepless nights caring for a newborn. But as days passed, her symptoms worsened. Simple tasks like climbing stairs or even breastfeeding left her gasping for air. She noticed her legs were unusually swollen, and her heart seemed to race even when she was resting. Alarmed, her husband rushed her to the emergency room.

From Newborn Bliss to Medical Emergency

The doctors immediately performed a physical examination and noted her rapid heart rate, low blood pressure and crackling sounds in her lungs, indicating fluid accumulation. Suspecting a cardiac issue, they ordered an echocardiogram. The results confirmed their fears: Ananya's heart's ejection fraction – a measure of how well the heart pumps blood – was only 30 per cent, far below the normal range of 55–70 per cent. She was diagnosed with peripartum cardiomyopathy, a rare but potentially life-threatening condition that weakens the heart muscle in late pregnancy or postpartum.

The news was devastating. Ananya had never imagined her heart could fail at a time that was supposed to be the happiest of her life. The doctors explained that this condition is uncommon, affecting 1 in 1,000 to 1 in 4,000 pregnancies, and its exact cause remains unclear. Risk factors include advanced maternal age, twin pregnancies and pre-eclampsia, none of which applied to her. It was glaring proof of how unpredictable life can be.

Understanding Peripartum Cardiomyopathy

Ananya's treatment began immediately. She was put on diuretics to reduce fluid build-up in her lungs and legs, beta-blockers to slow her heart rate and decrease the workload on her heart and angiotensin-converting enzyme (ACE) inhibitors (a type of medicine that regulates blood pressure) to improve her heart function. She was also advised to avoid another pregnancy as it could further strain her heart and prove fatal.

Over the following weeks, Ananya's condition slowly improved. Regular follow-ups showed her ejection fraction increasing to 45 per cent, a promising sign. Her cardiologist explained that with proper treatment, many women with this condition recover fully, though some may need lifelong heart medication.

The Importance of Maternal Heart Health

The experience changed Ananya's perspective on life. She became a defender for maternal heart health, sharing her story to raise awareness about peripartum cardiomyopathy. She urged women to listen to their bodies and seek medical attention if something feels wrong during or after pregnancy.

Ananya's journey was not without challenges, but her endurance and support system helped her sail through the rough waters. Holding her baby in her arms, she promised to cherish every moment and live each day to its fullest – a proof that a mother's heart stays strong, even in its weakest moments.

Peripartum cardiomyopathy is a rare condition but can have detrimental consequences. Early diagnosis and prompt treatment can save lives, highlighting the importance of awareness and timely medical care.

Gestational diabetes mellitus (GDM)

GDM is a type of diabetes that develops during pregnancy due to hormonal changes, insulin resistance and the increased metabolic demands of pregnancy. It usually occurs after the twenty-fourth week and resolves after delivery in most cases. However, it poses risks for both the mother and baby if left untreated.

Signs and Symptoms

GDM is often asymptomatic and detected through routine screening. However, some women may experience the following subtle signs:

1. Increased thirst and urination: Excess glucose in the blood pulls water into the kidneys, causing frequent urination and dehydration.
2. Fatigue: High blood sugar levels can impair the body's ability to use glucose for energy, leading to fatigue.
3. Blurred vision: Fluctuations in blood sugar can affect the lens of the eye, causing temporary blurriness.
4. Recurrent infections: Increased glucose levels can impair immune function, making women prone to urinary tract infections or yeast infections.
5. Excessive foetal growth (Macrosomia): Rapid or excessive foetal growth may signal uncontrolled blood sugar levels.

Risk Factors

1. Obesity or excessive weight gain during pregnancy
2. Family history of diabetes

3. Previous pregnancy with GDM
4. Advanced maternal age (more than thirty-five years)
5. Polycystic ovary syndrome
6. History of delivering a macrosomic baby (more than 4 kg)

Screening and Diagnosis

Screening for GDM is typically performed between twenty-four and twenty-eight weeks of gestation using:

1. Oral glucose tolerance test
   a. 50 g glucose challenge test: This is a non-fasting test. If plasma glucose is more than 140 mg/dL, a 3-hour oral glucose tolerance test is recommended.
   b. 100 g oral glucose tolerance test: This is a fasting test where blood sugar is measured at fasting, 1 hour, 2 hours and 3 hours. GDM is diagnosed if two or more values are elevated.
2. Fasting plasma glucose: A fasting glucose level of more than 92 mg/dL in the first trimester may also indicate GDM.

Management

Effective management is crucial to minimise complications such as macrosomia (a life-threatening condition that affects both the mother and the baby), preterm delivery and maternal diabetes postpartum.

Lifestyle Modifications

1. Dietary changes: Adopt a well-balanced diet with controlled carbohydrates, lean proteins and healthy fats. Avoid refined sugars and high-glycaemic foods.
2. Physical activity: Engage in moderate-intensity exercises (for example, walking, yoga) to improve insulin sensitivity.

Blood Sugar Monitoring

Frequent self-monitoring of blood glucose helps maintain glucose within target levels:

1. Fasting: less than 95 mg/dL
2. 1-hour postprandial: less than 140 mg/dL
3. 2-hour postprandial: less than 120 mg/dL

Medications

1. If lifestyle changes are insufficient, pharmacological treatment may be initiated.
2. Insulin is the preferred treatment as it does not cross the placenta.
3. Oral medications such as metformin or glyburide may be used as alternatives but are less commonly preferred.

Monitoring Foetal Health

1. Regular ultrasound scans must be done to monitor foetal growth, amniotic fluid levels and placental function.
2. Non-stress tests are done in the third trimester for high-risk cases.

Complications

Untreated GDM can lead to:

1. maternal risks such as pre-eclampsia, preterm labour and increased risk of type 2 diabetes postpartum and
2. foetal risks such as macrosomia, hypoglycaemia at birth, respiratory distress syndrome and long-term obesity or diabetes risk.

Postpartum Care

1. Blood sugar levels should be checked six to twelve weeks postpartum to rule out persistent diabetes.

2. Women with GDM are at increased risk of type 2 diabetes and should undergo regular glucose screenings.

With timely diagnosis and proper management, the risks associated with GDM can be minimised, ensuring a healthy pregnancy and delivery.

> 'Heart disease is not just an issue for South Asian men. A woman's lifetime risk of dying from heart disease is eight times greater than that of breast cancer! Heart disease in women has tragic consequences for families and society.'
> Indian Heart Association[1]

10

Beyond the Reps: Gym and Sudden Cardiac Deaths

Pushing the Limits

Akshay, a twenty-one-year-old gym enthusiast, lived for the iron. He spent hours sculpting his body, pushing limits most would not dare to touch. His workout ritual was a mix of heavy weights and caffeinated supplements, driven by the need to achieve the 'perfect physique'. However, one evening, his constant desire for perfection became a nightmare.

The Fatal Mix: Pre-Workout and Alcohol

After an intense leg-day session fuelled by a high-dose pre-workout supplement, Akshay joined his friends for a night out. The supplement – packed with caffeine, beta-alanine and stimulants – had already pushed his heart rate to its limit during exercise. Adding alcohol to the mix, a diuretic that disrupts electrolytes and promotes dehydration, was like throwing fuel on a smouldering fire.

Hours later, Akshay felt a racing heartbeat and a wave of dizziness. Before anyone could react, he collapsed, froth spilling from his mouth. His heart had entered ventricular fibrillation, a chaotic quivering of the heart's lower chambers that effectively stops blood pumping. Akshay was clinically dead for several minutes until paramedics arrived, performing CPR and shocking his heart back to life.

At the hospital, an angiogram revealed something shocking for someone his age: a 100 per cent blockage in his left anterior descending artery, commonly called the 'widowmaker'. This complete blockage led to a massive and almost fatal heart attack.

In recent years, pre-workout supplements have gained immense popularity among fitness enthusiasts seeking to boost energy, endurance and focus during their workouts. These supplements are designed to enhance performance by stimulating the body with a potent blend of ingredients like caffeine, amino acids and creatine. For many, the promise of increased energy and enhanced athletic performance is irresistible. However, while these supplements are marketed as a way to optimise workouts, the reality is that they come with potential dangers, particularly when misused or combined with other substances like alcohol. The risks associated with pre-workout supplements often go unnoticed until a serious incident occurs, as demonstrated by Akshay's life-threatening experience.

The Hidden Risks of Pre-Workout Supplements

Pre-workout supplements are a gym staple for many athletes, but they come with hidden dangers. Most are loaded with the following:

1. High doses of caffeine, which can cause rapid heart rate, increased blood pressure and palpitations, especially when combined with exercise
2. Beta-alanine and creatine, which, while safe in moderation, can lead to muscle cramps and dehydration in excess
3. Unregulated ingredients as many supplements contain hidden stimulants or banned substances

The combination of pre-workout supplements and alcohol amplifies risks, leading to severe dehydration, electrolyte imbalances and arrhythmias.

During his recovery, doctors learnt Akshay had also been using anabolic steroids (a synthetic steroid hormone that resembles testosterone) and testosterone injections to fast-track his muscle growth. These substances promise quick gains but come at a heavy cost.

The Steroid Trap: Building Muscles at a Deadly Cost

1. Heart damage: Steroids increase bad cholesterol (LDL) and decrease good cholesterol (high-density lipoprotein [HDL]), promoting the build-up of plaques in arteries like Akshay's left anterior descending artery.
2. High blood pressure: Chronic use of steroids causes hypertension and thickens the heart's left ventricle, reducing its efficiency.
3. Blood clots: Steroids promote clot formation, increasing the risk of heart attacks and strokes.
4. Arrhythmias: Steroids disrupt potassium, calcium and magnesium levels, increasing the risk of abnormal heart rhythms.

Testosterone misuse is another common pitfall. While medically indicated in some conditions, using it recklessly can suppress natural hormone production. Beta-human chorionic gonadotropin (beta-hCG), often used alongside testosterone to prevent testicular atrophy, should only be administered under medical guidance. Self-medicating with beta-hCG can lead to hormonal imbalances and further cardiac stress.

Target Heart Rate: An Important Realisation for Neo-Athletes

Akshay's obsession with performance meant he rarely paid attention to his target heart rate. New athletes often assume that pushing harder equals better results, but the truth is that the heart can only sustain so much.

For healthy exercise, individuals should aim for 70–85 per cent of their maximum heart rate (220 minus age). Surpassing this range, especially with stimulants like pre-workout supplements, increases the risk of overtraining, arrhythmias and cardiac arrest. Akshay's pre-workout had already pushed his heart rate dangerously high before the alcohol exacerbated the strain.

Advisory

Akshay survived due to timely CPR and advanced medical care, but the incident left him with stents in his left anterior descending artery and a lifetime of cardiac follow-ups. His journey serves as a grim reminder of the hidden dangers lurking in the fitness world.

Gym-goers must remember that fitness is about health, not shortcuts. Instead of relying on pre-workout supplements, steroids or testosterone for results, aspiring athletes should focus on balanced nutrition, consistent training and respect for their body's limits.

For those already using performance-enhancing drugs, seeking medical advice and monitoring cardiovascular health are essential. If testosterone therapy is prescribed, beta-hCG should only be taken under a doctor's supervision to maintain hormonal balance safely.

Expert Opinions on the Incident

1. Cardiologist's perspective: Dr Rajiv Sharma, a cardiologist, explained, 'Young individuals often underestimate the impact of energy drinks and pre-workouts on their heart. These stimulants elevate heart rate and blood pressure, which, when combined with alcohol, can lead to fatal arrhythmias or myocardial infarction.'[1]
2. Fitness trainer's view: A certified fitness trainer emphasised, 'Supplements should complement – not replace – a balanced diet. Many young gym-goers are unaware of their body's limits and push too hard, fuelled by these products.'

3. Role of education: Experts agree that gyms and supplement brands must educate consumers about the risks associated with overuse. Transparency in labelling and stringent regulatory oversight are also essential.

The Need for Change

Akshay's tragic story is not an isolated case. Reports of sudden deaths among fitness enthusiasts highlight the urgent need for greater awareness about heart health and safe fitness practices.

1. Screening programmes: Routine health screenings, including ECGs and stress tests, should be mandatory for young athletes, particularly those engaging in high-intensity training.
2. Regulation of supplements: Governments must enforce stricter regulations on dietary supplements to ensure they are free of harmful substances.
3. Community outreach: Fitness centres should conduct workshops on safe exercise practices, hydration and nutrition to foster a healthier gym culture.

The Learning

Akshay's story highlights a critical gap in awareness among young fitness enthusiasts: the heart is not invincible. Whether through unregulated supplements, steroids or overtraining, pushing too hard can lead to irreversible damage. Ultimately, fitness should be a journey to health – not a gamble with your life.

> Energy drinks can trigger heart problems. High caffeine and taurine levels can cause dangerous arrhythmias and sudden cardiac arrest.

11

Miracle at the Airport: When Time Was Running Out

A CEO's Fight for Life

Ramesh Mehta, a dynamic forty-five-year-old CEO, was known for his demanding schedule, often juggling work commitments while rushing between meetings and airports. One fateful morning, as he hurried to catch a flight to an international business conference, he collapsed unexpectedly in the airport lounge.

Passengers around him were completely shocked, unsure of what to do, until one individual stepped forward. A trained first responder, this good Samaritan recognised the gravity of the situation and immediately began performing CPR. The swift action kept blood flowing to Ramesh's brain and vital organs, buying precious time.

The Power of Automated External Defibrillators in Cardiac Emergencies

Within minutes, airport staff brought an automated external defibrillator (AED), a portable device designed to diagnose life-threatening heart rhythms and deliver an electric shock if necessary. The machine analysed Ramesh's heart rhythm and advised a shock, indicating that he was in ventricular fibrillation, a chaotic rhythm that prevents the heart from pumping blood effectively.

The bystander used the AED as instructed, delivering a shock that temporarily restored Ramesh's heart rhythm. By the time paramedics arrived, he had regained a weak pulse and was rushed to the nearest ER for advanced care.

Challenges in the ER: Recurrent Ventricular Tachycardia and Extracorporeal Membrane Oxygenation Support

At the hospital, Ramesh's condition remained critical. He suffered recurrent episodes of ventricular tachycardia, a dangerous arrhythmia (irregular heartbeat) that can lead to cardiac arrest. Despite anti-arrhythmic medications and advanced life support, his heart continued to struggle.

Given his worsening condition, the medical team decided to place him on extracorporeal membrane oxygenation, a life-saving machine that temporarily took over the function of his heart and lungs. This support allowed his heart to rest and recover while ensuring that oxygenated blood circulated throughout his body.

After 48 hours on the machine, his cardiac function stabilised, and the team weaned him off it. However, the underlying risk of life-threatening arrhythmias persisted, necessitating a long-term solution.

The Role of an ICD

To prevent future episodes of sudden cardiac arrest, the doctors implanted an ICD. This small device monitors heart rhythms continuously and delivers a shock if it detects an abnormal rhythm like ventricular fibrillation or ventricular tachycardia.

For someone like Ramesh, the device would act as a safety net, significantly reducing the risk of sudden cardiac death. He was discharged a few days later, thankful to be alive and determined to spread awareness about the importance of timely intervention.

Importance of CPR, AEDs and ICDs

Ramesh's narrative highlights three critical aspects of surviving cardiac arrest.

1. CPR training saves lives: CPR is the foundation of emergency response for cardiac arrest. Chest compressions keep blood flowing to vital organs, increasing the chances of survival until professional help arrives. Every individual, regardless of their profession, should learn basic CPR techniques. Public training programmes can empower bystanders to act swiftly and confidently.
2. Widespread availability of AEDs: An AED is a life-saving device that is simple to use, even by those without medical training. Many public spaces, including airports, malls and stadiums, now have AEDs, but awareness and accessibility remain challenges. A combination of CPR and AED usage dramatically improves survival rates in cardiac arrest cases.
3. Importance of an ICD: Patients at high risk for life-threatening arrhythmias benefit greatly from an ICD. This device provides continuous monitoring and instant intervention, acting as a guardian against sudden cardiac death. Advances in ICD technology have made these devices more reliable and patient-friendly, with minimal risk during implantation.

A Wake-Up Call

Ramesh's near-death experience emphasises the importance of public preparedness for cardiac emergencies. Quick thinking by a bystander trained in CPR, access to an AED and timely hospital intervention gave him a second chance at life. As Ramesh recovered, he became an advocate for promoting CPR training and increasing AED availability in public spaces. His company even sponsored free CPR workshops and donated AEDs to schools and community centres. In Ramesh's words, 'I owe my life to a stranger who knew CPR, an AED at the airport and the team that gave me a second heart with the ICD. Every second mattered that day, and it made all the difference.'

The Learning

Sudden cardiac arrest can happen to anyone, anywhere. By equipping ourselves with knowledge and ensuring access to life-saving tools, we can turn bystanders into heroes and give more people like Ramesh a fighting chance. Every heartbeat matters, and every life is worth saving.

CPR is often done wrong. Most bystanders don't push hard or fast enough.

The Right Way to Do CPR

1. Push 2 inches deep
2. 100–120 compressions per minute (like the beat of 'Stayin' Alive')
3. No mouth-to-mouth needed, just chest compressions.

12

Unpacking Obesity: The Struggles, Science and Sustainable Solutions

Mr Singh, a forty-five-year-old office worker, weighs 120 kg with a BMI of 35, placing him in the obese category. His sedentary lifestyle, unhealthy eating habits and lack of structured exercise have contributed to his weight gain over the years. His complaints of fatigue, joint pain and breathlessness highlight the physical toll of obesity. However, these symptoms are just the tip of the iceberg as obesity increases his risk for cardiovascular disease, diabetes and hypertension.

The Thrifty Gene Hypothesis

Obesity is not merely the result of overeating and lack of exercise. The 'thrifty gene' hypothesis suggests that our ancestors developed a genetic tendency to efficiently store fat as an energy reserve during times of famine. In today's environment, where food is abundant, this genetic trait predisposes individuals to store excess fat, contributing to obesity.

Subcutaneous Fat versus Visceral Fat

Subcutaneous fat is stored under the skin. It accounts for the majority of body fat and is relatively less harmful. Visceral fat is stored around internal organs like the liver, the heart and the intestines. It actively secretes pro-inflammatory hormones, increasing the risk of type 2 diabetes, CAD and fatty liver.

Fat Metabolism and Obesity Challenges

Fat metabolism is the process where the body breaks down fat to use for energy. This happens when the body turns stored fat (called triglycerides) into fatty acids, which are then used as fuel. However, when someone is overweight for a long time, their body can start resisting fat loss. This is because of hormonal imbalances, such as resistance to leptin, a hormone that helps control hunger and fat storage. When the body becomes resistant to these hormones, it makes it much harder to lose weight, even with diet and exercise.

While the body has natural mechanisms for burning fat, achieving lasting weight loss is not always straightforward. Many people turn to quick fixes, such as crash diets, in an attempt to shed excess weight quickly. However, while these diets may show rapid results in the short term, they often fail to address the root causes of weight gain and can lead to harmful long-term effects. Instead of focusing on sustainable lifestyle changes, crash diets often create more problems than they solve, making it harder to maintain weight loss over time.

Why Do Crash Diets Fail?

1. Muscle loss: Extreme calorie restriction prioritises burning muscle for energy, slowing metabolism.
2. Nutrient deficiencies: Lack of essential vitamins and minerals leads to fatigue and weakened immunity.
3. Rebound weight gain: Post-diet overeating often leads to regaining more weight than was initially lost.

Common Crash Diets

1. Juice cleanses, often nutrient-deficient, lead to quick weight loss but no fat loss.
2. Very low-calorie diets may trigger metabolic slowdown and unsustainable results.

When it comes to weight loss, there's no one-size-fits-all solution. While quick-fix diets can offer temporary results, a sustainable approach is key to achieving long-term health and maintaining weight loss. The best diets are those that are balanced, flexible and suitable for your personal lifestyle, preferences and health needs. Understanding the different types of diets available can help you choose one that supports not only your weight loss goals but also your overall well-being.

Types of Diets

Ketogenic Diet

1. This diet is high in fats and very low in carbs.
2. It is effective for quick weight loss but difficult to maintain.
3. The risks include keto flu and nutrient deficiencies.

Intermittent Fasting

1. Eating windows (for example, 16:8) encourage calorie control.
2. The benefits are improved insulin sensitivity and digestion.
3. It may lead to binge eating if not managed.

Mediterranean Diet

1. Focus on olive oil, nuts, lean protein and fresh produce.
2. This diet is proven to improve heart health and sustain weight loss.

DASH (Dietary Approaches to Stop Hypertension) Diet

Originally for hypertension management, it focuses on fruits, vegetables and whole grains.

A Sustainable Weight Loss Approach

By focusing on long-term goals, individuals can adopt sustainable practices that support gradual weight loss, enhance overall well-being and promote a balanced lifestyle. This approach encourages mindful eating, regular physical activity and informed food choices that align with personal preferences and nutritional needs, ultimately leading to lasting results and a healthier life.

Key Principles

1. Caloric deficit: Achieve weight loss by burning more calories than consumed.
2. Balanced macros: This dietary strategy ensures a healthy balance among all three nutritional categories by distributing the intake of macronutrients – carbohydrates, proteins and fats – in a precise, well-proportioned ratio to match individual needs.
   a. Carbohydrates: 45–50 per cent (opt for whole grains, fruits and vegetables).
   b. Protein: 20–25 per cent (lean meats, tofu and legumes).
   c. Fats: 25–30 per cent (healthy sources like avocado, nuts and olive oil).
3. Consistency: Small, gradual changes in dietary habits and lifestyle are more effective for achieving long-term weight loss and maintaining a healthy weight.
4. Behavioural strategies:
   a. Mindful eating: Slow down, savour your meals and recognise satiety cues.
   b. Food journalling: It helps identify triggers and track progress.
   c. Sleep: At least 7–8 hours of sleep is required to optimise metabolism and reduce cravings.
   d. Stress management: Yoga, meditation or therapy can combat emotional eating.

Practical Weight Loss Plan

You can follow this easy diet plan that can help you achieve lasting results without any harmful effects.

Breakfast (7:30 AM)

Two boiled eggs or one bowl of oatmeal with chia seeds and berries

Mid-morning Snack (10:30 AM)

One handful of nuts (almonds or walnuts)

Lunch (1:00 PM)

1. Grilled chicken breast or paneer
2. One cup of steamed broccoli and carrots
3. One small portion of quinoa or brown rice

Evening Snack (4:30 PM)

One cup of green tea with one fruit (for example, apple or pear)

Dinner (7:30 PM)

1. Baked fish or lentil soup
2. Salad with olive oil dressing
3. One whole-grain roti or a small bowl of dal
4. Hydration: 2–3 litres of water per day

Physical Activity

1. Start with 30 minutes of brisk walking daily, progressing to strength training and cardio exercises.
2. Incorporate flexibility exercises like yoga once a week.

Monitoring and Adjustment

1. Weekly weigh-ins: Track progress but don't obsess over daily fluctuations.
2. Diet adjustments: Modify portions or calorie intake as weight loss plateaus.
3. Medical support: Consider metabolic studies or supervised weight-loss programmes if needed.

The Learning

Obesity management is complex but achievable with a tailored approach combining scientific understanding, consistent effort and a sustainable lifestyle. Crash diets and quick fixes may promise results but often lead to disappointment. A long-term focus on balanced nutrition, physical activity and behavioural change is key to unlocking better health and quality of life.

> Heartburn and a heart attack can feel the same. If your 'acidity' is new, severe or occurs with sweating and breathlessness, it could be a heart attack.

13

Stress Testing Your Heart: A Vital Step for Busy Executives

STRESS ECHOCARDIOGRAPHY AND cardiopulmonary exercise testing are important tools that help doctors find heart problems, especially in people who may not show any obvious symptoms. Sometimes, regular health check-ups can uncover serious issues, allowing doctors to step in before things get worse. This chapter looks at the story of Rajesh Mehta, a forty-five-year-old executive who found out about a dangerous heart blockage thanks to routine testing.

What is Stress Echocardiography?

Stress echocardiography is a method that uses ultrasound to see how well your heart works under stress, either from exercise or medication. It helps identify areas where blood flow may be reduced, which can be a sign of CAD. There are two main types of stress echocardiography:

1. Exercise stress echocardiography: The patient works out on a treadmill or a stationary bike while images of the heart are taken before and after the exercise.
2. Dobutamine stress echocardiography: If someone can't exercise, a medication called dobutamine is used to mimic exercise effects by raising the heart rate.

Both methods are non-invasive and help to assess how well the heart is functioning.

Cardiopulmonary Exercise Testing

This is a comprehensive test that looks at how your heart, lungs and muscles respond when you exercise. It measures things like oxygen usage and carbon dioxide output, giving a clearer picture of your exercise capacity. This test is particularly helpful for:

1. understanding unexplained shortness of breath or difficulty exercising,
2. evaluating risks for people with known or suspected heart issues and
3. checking how patients with heart failure are responding to treatment.

The Case of the Executive

Rajesh Mehta was a busy CEO who decided to get a routine health check-up due to work stress. Despite leading a seemingly healthy life, he sometimes felt fatigued, which he blamed on his hectic schedule. As part of his check-up, his doctor suggested stress echocardiography and cardiopulmonary exercise testing to assess his cardiopulmonary fitness.

The Testing Process

Step 1

Resting echocardiography: The first echocardiogram showed that Rajesh's heart function was normal.

Step 2

Stress testing: During the exercise test on the treadmill, doctors noticed some irregularities in his heart's electrical activity at peak exertion, hinting at a possible heart issue.

After Rajesh completed the exercise stress test, doctors used echocardiography to look at how his heart was functioning. The tests indicated that some parts of his heart were not getting enough oxygen-rich blood, which could lead to serious heart issues. These findings were important because they pointed to potential problems with his heart's blood supply.

Step 3

Cardiopulmonary exercise testing: During this test, doctors made several important observations about Rajesh's heart and lung function while he exercised.

1. First, they found that his VO_2max, which is the maximum amount of oxygen his body can use during intense exercise, was lower than expected. So his body wasn't getting enough oxygen when he was active, which is a sign that not all parts of his body were receiving good blood flow.
2. They also noticed something called an early anaerobic threshold. This term means that Rajesh's body started to struggle with providing enough oxygen before reaching the usual point in exercise. This suggests that his heart was having difficulties pumping blood effectively when he exerted himself, indicating that it wasn't functioning at its best during physical activity.
3. Finally, they measured the respiratory exchange ratio, which looks at how well his body was exchanging oxygen and carbon dioxide during exercise. This result came back normal, meaning Rajesh's lungs seemed to be working fine and didn't show any immediate signs of problems related to breathing.

Step 4

Dobutamine stress echocardiography: Because the earlier test results were somewhat concerning but not definitive, doctors decided to perform a dobutamine stress echocardiography to get clearer answers. In this test, they gradually increased the dose of a medication called dobutamine, which acts like exercise for the heart. At a specific dose of 40 micrograms per kilogram per minute, Rajesh began to show changes in how his heart was working.

1. The images taken during this test showed that the same areas of the heart that had trouble moving earlier continued to show signs of problems, confirming that there were issues in those parts of the heart.
2. Additionally, they noticed a drop in blood pressure during this test, which further indicated that he might have significant blockages in the arteries supplying blood to his heart. This drop in blood pressure, along with the earlier findings, reinforced the concern that Rajesh had serious issues related to his heart health.

Diagnostic Conclusion

Based on all the tests and results, doctors strongly believed that Rajesh had a serious blockage in the arteries that supply blood to his heart. Because of this concern, he was sent for a specialised test called coronary angiography. This test showed that one of his arteries, specifically the proximal right coronary artery, was blocked by 90 per cent. Only a small amount of blood could flow through that artery, which is very dangerous for his heart.

Understanding the Results

Why Stress Echo Was Key

The stress echocardiography test was essential because it showed that some parts of Rajesh's heart weren't moving properly when under stress. This helped doctors figure out exactly which areas of the heart were affected by poor blood flow. In Rajesh's case, the problems were found in the inferior and posterior parts of the heart, which matched the findings of the blockage in the right coronary artery.

Cardiopulmonary Exercise Testing's Role in Risk Assessment

The test results indicated that Rajesh's body used less oxygen than expected during exercise. This suggested that his heart wasn't working as well as it should be, which meant further tests were necessary. The results worked together with the stress echo findings, providing a complete view of how well Rajesh's heart and lungs were functioning.

Importance of Dobutamine Stress Echo

The dobutamine stress echo was performed to double-check the previous findings, especially since Rajesh had some trouble with exercise intensity. This test confirmed that he indeed had areas of reduced blood flow, or ischaemia, in the same parts of his heart that the other tests pointed out.

Management of CAD

Immediate Treatments

Following these tests, Rajesh underwent a procedure called percutaneous coronary intervention, where a small tube, or stent, was placed in the right coronary artery. This helped open the blocked artery, restoring normal blood flow to his heart and significantly lowering his chances of having a heart attack in the future.

Lifestyle Modifications

After the procedure, Rajesh's doctor stressed the importance of making some lifestyle changes to keep his heart healthy. This included the following:

- Following a diet rich in vegetables, fruits and whole grains and low in saturated fats and sugar
- Practising methods to manage stress, such as yoga and mindfulness exercises
- Attending regular health check-ups to keep an eye on his cholesterol levels and blood pressure

Long-Term Medical Treatment

Rajesh was also prescribed a combination of medications. He was given dual antiplatelet therapy (two different medications, aspirin and clopidogrel) to help prevent blood clots, a statin (atorvastatin) to lower cholesterol levels and a beta-blocker to help his heart work more efficiently and prevent future problems.

Broader Implications

Why Routine Testing Matters

Rajesh's case highlights how important it is for everyone, especially busy professionals, to have regular health check-ups. Sometimes people don't know they have heart issues because they might not feel any pain or symptoms. If these issues go unnoticed, they can lead to serious problems like a heart attack.

Advancements in Non-Invasive Testing

Modern advancements in stress echo and cardiopulmonary exercise testing have improved the accuracy of these tests, making them even better at finding heart problems early. New methods like special imaging techniques that look at heart muscle movement can help catch blockages even sooner.

Role of Comprehensive Screening

Having a thorough approach to heart health is vital. Combining stress tests, cardiopulmonary exercise testing and advanced imaging can help doctors identify people at high risk for heart problems before they start experiencing any symptoms.

The Learning

Rajesh Mehta's experience shows just how important routine testing is for catching hidden heart issues. The stress echocardiography, cardiopulmonary exercise testing and dobutamine stress echo tests played crucial roles in diagnosing his heart condition and guiding timely medical action. For busy individuals, his story is a reminder that ignoring subtle signs or skipping regular health appointments can lead to severe health consequences. Taking an active approach to heart health assessments is essential for preventing heart disease and living long, healthy lives. With rising risks of heart problems among younger people, integrating advanced non-invasive diagnostics into regular health check-ups is not just helpful but necessary.

> Watching sports can trigger a heart attack. Intense emotional stress (like watching your team lose) can spike blood pressure and trigger arrhythmias.

14

From Health to Hospital: A Fit Life Takes a Sudden Twist

AT FORTY-SEVEN, VIKRAM WAS the picture of health. He was athletic, didn't smoke and loved running over 10 kilometres every other day. His days were filled with energy and balance, making him feel unstoppable. So when he suddenly noticed he was a bit short of breath after a 5-kilometre run, he didn't think much of it. After all, he had enjoyed some treats at a family wedding and hadn't been sleeping well. So he figured it was just a temporary issue.

Determined to get back on track, Vikram laced up his running shoes for another run the next morning. However, this time, something felt off. He experienced a vague pain between his shoulder blades. It was odd but not intense enough to stop his run. After he got home, he took an antacid for his discomfort and rested for a bit. Feeling slightly better, he decided to drive from Faridabad to his office in Gurgaon, pushing the strange feelings to the back of his mind.

Later that day, a security guard called Vikram to warn him about a tree that was about to fall on his car due to heavy rain and storms. Alarmed, Vikram hurried downstairs to move his car. Since the lift was busy, he quickly took the stairs from his office on the sixth floor. As he reached his car and was about to grab his keys, something frightening happened – he suddenly felt a lack of air, became light-headed and then collapsed right there on the ground.

CPR Can Make All the Difference

Initially, bystanders thought he had slipped due to the rain. However, when he didn't get back up after a few minutes, the security guard realised this was serious. Luckily, some of Vikram's colleagues had just completed a CPR course and were trained in basic life support. They rushed to help him, immediately starting CPR, and took him to the hospital emergency room.

Vikram was put on a ventilator, and a team of heart specialists was called in. Within moments, he was in the catheterisation lab for an urgent angiography. The doctors discovered something shocking – a 100 per cent blockage in his left anterior descending artery. This artery plays a vital role in supplying blood to the heart. The doctors quickly removed the clot using a technique called thrombosuction and performed coronary angioplasty to restore blood flow.

In a surprising turn of events, Vikram woke up the next day and was taken off the ventilator. Remarkably, he was able to go home just 48 hours later.

Important Lessons Learnt

1. Trust your body: Subtle signs, such as unexpected shortness of breath or odd pain, should not be ignored. Even someone like Vikram, with no known health risks, was experiencing serious issues. His body was sending him warning signals that he should have paid attention to.
2. The importance of CPR: The quick response from his CPR-trained colleagues was crucial in saving Vikram's life. If they hadn't acted quickly and performed CPR, he might not have made it to the hospital.
3. Family health screening is important: Despite his seemingly perfect health, Vikram was found to have a genetic condition called heterozygous familial hypercholesterolaemia, which causes high cholesterol levels. Doctors recommended that his family, especially his two sons aged nineteen and thirteen, should get screened to catch any potential issues

early. Sadly, they declined to have the tests done, fearing that it would bring social stigma and make it harder for the boys to get married in the future.
4. Stay ahead with testing: Vikram's case shows that even without obvious risk factors, it is wise to undergo tests such as a computed tomography (CT) coronary calcium score or a thorough cholesterol check. These tests can help identify individuals who are at high risk for heart disease before serious problems arise.

Simple Breakdown of Cholesterol

Cholesterol often gets divided into two main types: LDL, known as 'bad' cholesterol, and HDL, referred to as 'good' cholesterol. LDL can build up in blood vessels, leading to dangerous blockages like the one Vikram faced, while HDL helps to remove LDL from the bloodstream. In Vikram's case, his high LDL levels went unnoticed because he seemed otherwise healthy.

This story serves as a powerful wake-up call. It illustrates how crucial it is to recognise and act on early symptoms of health problems. Additionally, it underscores the life-saving importance of knowing CPR and being prepared to use it when necessary. Lastly, it highlights the significance of family health awareness and genetic screening, even amid societal fears of stigma.

Remember, taking care of your heart is vital. Listen to your body, stay informed about your family history and don't hesitate to seek medical advice if something feels off. Staying proactive about health can make all the difference in preventing heart-related emergencies and ensuring a long, healthy life.

> Being fit doesn't guarantee a healthy heart. Even athletes can have heart disease if they have genetic risks, high stress or bad sleep habits.

15

Heart Attack After Surgery

Balancing Health Risks

The intersection of surgical and cardiovascular care is a delicate balancing act. This story showcases a sad but preventable situation: a fifty-six-year-old man who suffered a severe heart attack after undergoing hernia surgery because he stopped taking his antiplatelet medications. This highlights the importance of consulting heart specialists before surgery and the dangers of stopping blood thinner medications without proper guidance.

The Patient's Journey: A Series of Events

Our story revolves around a fifty-six-year-old man. Just a month earlier, he had received two special stents in his heart arteries to help with blood flow after a heart attack. After getting these stents, his doctors prescribed dual antiplatelet therapy, which means he needed to take aspirin along with another heart medication to prevent blood clots.

He visited a surgeon complaining of worsening pain in his groin and was diagnosed with an inguinal hernia that needed surgery. Unfortunately, the surgeon told him to stop his heart medication five days before the surgery without consulting his cardiologist.

The surgery went well, or so it seemed. However, within a day, the patient began to experience severe chest pain, trouble breathing and a rapid decline in vital signs. He was rushed to the ICU, where an ECG confirmed that he was having a massive heart attack due to a blocked stent – an event likely caused by discontinuation of antiplatelets.

Why Stopping Heart Medications Is Risky

After stent placement, the body begins to heal. However, this healing process takes time, and the stent needs protection from blood clots during this phase. Antiplatelet medications are essential because they help prevent platelets (a type of blood cell) from sticking together and forming clots.

Early Stent Thrombosis

The most dangerous time for a heart stent is usually within the first month after placement. If a patient stops their antiplatelet medications too early, the risk of forming a blood clot around the stent increases significantly.

Surgical Risks

Any type of surgery can cause changes in blood flow and increase the chances of blood clots forming, especially if blood thinner medications are stopped.

The Importance of Multidisciplinary Communication

This case highlights a glaring gap in communication. The decision to stop antiplatelets was made without consulting the patient's cardiologist, reflecting a lack of interdisciplinary coordination. Several strategies could have prevented this catastrophic event:

1. Cardiology consultation: A discussion with the heart doctor before surgery could have clarified whether it was safe to continue the heart medications and assessed the risks of bleeding versus clotting.

2. Assessing risks: Patients with recent stent placements are at higher risk of blood clots. If possible, they should delay elective surgeries until it is safe to change the regimen of the heart medications, typically after six to twelve months.
3. Using alternative medications: If surgery is necessary, doctors could use other medications that help prevent clotting for a short time.

The Balancing Act: Bleeding versus Thrombosis

Stopping heart medications raises the risk of blood clots, while continuing them during surgery could lead to excessive bleeding. However, numerous studies reveal that the consequences of a blood clot (like a major heart attack or death) are far worse than the risks associated with surgical bleeding, which doctors can usually manage.

Supporting Evidence

The POISE-2 study indicates that continuing aspirin during the perioperative period does not significantly increase major bleeding risks, reinforcing the idea that it should be kept on schedule for high-risk patients.[1]

Timing of Surgery Post-Stenting

If a patient has had a stent placed in their artery to keep it open, they should wait before undergoing non-emergency or elective surgery. The waiting period depends on the type of stent. For bare-metal stents, at least thirty days should pass before elective surgery, and for drug-eluting stents, ideally, six to twelve months should elapse before elective surgery. This delay is recommended to reduce the risk of blood clots (stent thrombosis) and other complications as stopping blood-thinning medications too soon after stenting can be dangerous.

Recommended Guidelines for Managing Antiplatelet Therapy Before Surgery

Leading medical organisations like the American College of Cardiology and the European Society of Cardiology provide clear recommendations on how to handle heart medications before surgery:[2]

1. Delay non-urgent surgeries: Whenever possible, postpone non-emergency surgeries until patients can safely stop dual antiplatelet therapy.
2. Keep aspirin during surgery: Generally, patients should continue taking aspirin unless their risk of bleeding is extremely high.
3. Restart medication quickly: If there is a need to interrupt antiplatelet therapy for surgery, it should be resumed as soon as bleeding is controlled.

A Helpful Checklist for Doctors

Before Surgery

1. Get a complete heart health history, including any recent stent procedures.
2. Consult a heart specialist for patients at high risk.
3. Discuss the pros and cons of stopping or continuing heart medications.

During Surgery

1. Use careful surgical techniques to minimise bleeding.
2. Consider regional anaesthesia, which can help reduce blood loss.

After Surgery

1. Monitor patients closely for signs of heart issues or bleeding complications.
2. Restart antiplatelet therapy as soon as it is safe to do so.

The Aftermath: A Preventable Tragedy

Despite immediate medical intervention, including an emergency procedure to reopen the blocked stent, the patient faced many complications. His recovery was challenging, with issues like heart dysfunction and a prolonged stay in the ICU. This tragic outcome was avoidable with better planning and communication before the surgery.

Key Takeaways from This Case

1. Consulting a cardiologist is important. Any patient with a recent history of stent placement should have a thorough preoperative assessment by a heart specialist to ensure their heart health is prioritised.
2. Antiplatelet medications are essential. Taking heart medications on time is critical. Stopping them too soon can lead to serious problems, including stent thrombosis.
3. Team collaboration is key. Surgeons, anaesthesiologists and cardiologists must work together to provide the best care for patients, ensuring all risks are adequately assessed and addressed.

Empowering Patients: Knowledge Is Power

Patients should be informed about the significance of adhering to prescribed medication regimens and the potential dangers of discontinuing their medications without professional advice. When patients understand their treatment plans, they can better advocate for themselves and ensure that all their healthcare providers are aware of their crucial medical histories.

The Learning

This case serves as a powerful reminder of the risks of neglecting the involvement of heart specialists in surgical care. The unfortunate heart attack that happened after a routine hernia procedure underscores the need to continue necessary heart medications, seek cardiology input before surgery and encourage teamwork among medical professionals. By following established guidelines and prioritising effective communication, healthcare providers can significantly reduce the risk of similar tragedies and improve outcomes for their patients.

> Dental health affects heart health. Poor oral hygiene increases inflammation and the risk of heart valve infections and blockages.

16

Blue Babies and an Asymptomatic Adult

CONGENITAL HEART DEFECTS, OFTEN referred to as 'holes in the heart', can manifest in different ways. Some are detected early in infancy due to noticeable symptoms, while others remain unnoticed until adulthood. In this chapter, we explore the varied experiences of individuals with structural heart conditions, the diverse ways these defects present and the differing approaches to treatment and observation.

Recognising Signs of Heart Trouble in Newborns

When a newborn baby turns blue while crying or sweats a lot during feeding, parents might think it is just a normal reaction. However, these signs can mean that there's something wrong with the baby's heart.

Case 1: Understanding the Signs

Take the case of little Aarav, born a healthy baby boy weighing 3.5 kilograms. His parents noticed something odd when he cried: his lips and skin would turn slightly blue, but once he calmed down, the colour returned to normal. They also realised that Aarav would sweat excessively while breastfeeding, leaving his tiny head damp after each feed. Initially, they thought it was because of the effort Aarav put into feeding or crying, but during a routine check-up, the paediatrician raised concerns and recommended further testing.

Aarav was diagnosed with a congenital heart defect, a condition present from birth where the heart doesn't form correctly. His blue lips during crying were due to poor oxygenation, and the sweating while feeding was a sign that his heart was working too hard to pump blood through his body.

In newborns, these subtle signs – turning blue (cyanosis) and sweating excessively – are often early indicators of heart problems. The heart may not be able to pump efficiently, and the oxygen supply to the body may be compromised. For babies like Aarav, timely diagnosis and treatment can be life-saving.

Aarav's parents, guided by their doctors, opted for a surgical procedure to correct his heart defect. After the surgery, Aarav recovered beautifully. He no longer turned blue when he cried, and feeding became much easier and more comfortable for him.

If your baby exhibits signs like blue lips or excessive sweating, especially during feeding or crying, it is important to consult a paediatrician right away. Early detection can make all the difference in ensuring your baby grows up healthy and strong.

Case 2: The Boy Who Conquered a Heart Condition

Arjun, a four-year-old boy, was born with tetralogy of Fallot, a complex congenital heart defect. From birth, his parents noticed his lips and fingertips often turned blue, especially when he cried or exerted himself. As he grew older, Arjun experienced 'Tet spells', where he would suddenly squat down during play. These spells, characterised by severe breathlessness, cyanosis and fatigue, were terrifying for his parents.

Tet spells occur when oxygen-poor blood flows into the body due to the heart's inability to pump oxygen-rich blood effectively. Arjun's doctor explained that he needed surgery to fix his heart, but his parents worried about the outcome. At the age of five, Arjun finally underwent surgery to repair the holes in his heart and open up the narrow blood vessel to his lungs. Although recovering was not easy, Arjun's strength and determination were inspiring.

Today, Arjun is a lively ten-year-old who plays football with his friends, attends school regularly and dreams of becoming a pilot. His parents ensure regular follow-ups with his cardiologist, and apart from minor activity modifications, he leads a completely normal life. Arjun's story illustrates how essential early treatment and medical advancements can be in addressing congenital heart conditions.

Case 3: A Tragic Tale of Delay in Care

Ritika's story is tragically different. She was born with a small ventricular septal defect (VSD), a hole in the wall separating the two lower chambers of the heart. The size of the defect affects blood flow: with a large VSD, blood flows back into the lungs, increasing pressure and leading to heart failure if untreated. Her parents were told the hole in her heart might close on its own. At first, Ritika showed no symptoms and grew like any other child. But by the time she turned ten, subtle signs of fatigue, breathlessness and blue-tinged lips began to emerge.

Unfortunately, Ritika's family lived in a remote village with limited access to specialised healthcare. Her parents believed the symptoms were a phase she would outgrow, unaware that her condition was deteriorating. Over the years, the excessive blood flow to her lungs, caused by the uncorrected VSD, led to irreversible damage to the pulmonary arteries. By the time Ritika was properly diagnosed, she had developed Eisenmenger syndrome.

Now eighteen, Ritika's lips are permanently blue, and her stamina is severely limited. Even walking a short distance leaves her gasping for air. Her doctors explained that surgery is no longer an option due to the advanced stage of pulmonary hypertension. Ritika's condition is now managed with medications, including pulmonary vasodilators and diuretics, to control symptoms. However, her future remains uncertain.

Unlike Arjun's uplifting story, Ritika's case is an example of the devastating consequences of delayed diagnosis and treatment. The preventable progression of her VSD into Eisenmenger syndrome serves as a cautionary tale about the importance of timely medical intervention and regular follow-ups.

Case 4: A Young Child with Sweating

Arjun, a one-year-old, was brought to the paediatrician with symptoms that worried his parents: he would break into a sweat during feeds and seemed tired after only a few minutes of sucking. He struggled to gain weight, and his mother described him as 'always a bit frail' compared to other kids his age. Upon examination, the paediatrician noticed a murmur and ordered an echocardiogram, which confirmed a VSD.

Symptoms and Signs

Sweating during feeds, difficulty feeding, failure to thrive and tachypnoea (fast breathing) are common in infants with large VSDs. Arjun's symptoms matched this picture, indicating the need for immediate medical attention.

Types of VSDs

VSDs can range from small to large. Small VSDs (restrictive) are often asymptomatic and may close on their own during the first few years of life. These typically do not require treatment but need monitoring. Moderate to large VSDs typically cause symptoms of heart failure in infants and need medical management or surgical intervention.

Since Arjun's VSD was large, the paediatric cardiologist recommended surgery to close the hole. Medications such as diuretics may temporarily help reduce symptoms, but surgery or catheter-based intervention is usually essential for larger VSDs in young children. After successful surgery, Arjun's symptoms gradually improved, and he began gaining weight, catching up with milestones.

Case 5: The Asymptomatic Adult with Atrial Septal Defect (ASD)

Priya, a thirty-year-old woman, had lived her life without any noticeable heart-related symptoms. She had no history of fatigue, shortness of breath or other concerns and had recently visited her doctor for a routine check-up. However, her physician detected a heart murmur, prompting further investigation.

An echocardiogram revealed an ASD. ASD is a hole in the wall between the two upper chambers of the heart. Unlike VSD, ASD often remains asymptomatic in childhood and may go undetected until adulthood, as was the case with Priya.

Types of ASDs

Small ASDs are generally asymptomatic and often close on their own by early childhood. They typically do not require intervention but need occasional follow-up. Moderate to large ASDs may remain asymptomatic for years but can lead to complications in adulthood, such as arrhythmias, heart failure or pulmonary hypertension if untreated. Secundum ASD, the most common type, located in the middle of the atrial septum, often goes undiagnosed and may be detected incidentally.

Although Priya had no symptoms, her ASD was large enough that it posed a future risk. The cardiologist recommended a minimally invasive catheter-based procedure to close the defect. This is often preferable for adults with ASDs as it reduces future risks of heart complications. In cases with smaller defects, monitoring every few years without intervention may be sufficient.

Types of Heart Defects and Treatment Decisions

In children and adults, congenital heart defects vary in severity, location and the urgency for treatment. Some key types include:

1. VSD: As seen in Arjun, these defects can present with symptoms early in life. Small VSDs may close on their

own, while moderate to large VSDs usually require surgical closure, especially if there are symptoms of heart failure.
2. ASD: As seen in Priya, ASDs may go unnoticed for years and often remain asymptomatic. Small ASDs can close naturally, but larger ASDs should be closed, typically in adulthood, to prevent long-term complications.
3. Patent ductus arteriosus: This is a common congenital defect where the ductus arteriosus (a temporary vessel present in foetuses) fails to close after birth. Small defects may close on their own, but large ones can cause heart failure and should be treated.
4. Types of defects that usually don't need treatment: Small VSDs and small ASDs often close naturally, needing only routine monitoring. Small patent ductus arteriosus may also close on their own without treatment.

The Importance of Early Detection and Monitoring

These cases highlight the range of presentations for congenital heart defects. Symptoms like sweating during feeds, failure to thrive or fatigue should prompt investigation in infants as they often point to significant heart issues. For adults, incidental findings of murmurs or a family history of heart disease are reasons to consider a thorough evaluation as many defects, such as ASDs, may go undetected without symptoms.

For parents and individuals alike, understanding the types of heart defects, monitoring progress and being aware of symptoms can be life-saving. Early detection and appropriate treatment, whether surgery in childhood or a catheter procedure in adulthood, can improve outcomes and prevent complications, allowing patients to lead healthier lives.

Turning Blue: Understanding Eisenmenger Syndrome in Older Adults

It is not every day that we see an older person's lips, fingertips or face turn blue – cyanosis. Yet, for some people, this startling symptom is a sign of a rare and complex heart condition called Eisenmenger syndrome.

What Is Eisenmenger Syndrome?

Eisenmenger syndrome typically develops from untreated congenital heart defects, like a hole between the heart chambers (commonly a VSD). This defect can cause blood to flow abnormally, leading to too much blood in the lungs, which damages the lung's blood vessels over time. As resistance in the lungs increases, the pressure rises to a dangerous level, resulting in poorly oxygenated blood being pumped back into the body.

Although this condition typically develops in younger individuals, advances in healthcare mean that some patients may survive into their later years. For elderly patients, however, Eisenmenger syndrome often presents unique challenges.

Signs and Symptoms

The hallmark symptom of Eisenmenger syndrome is cyanosis, caused by low oxygen levels in the blood. This can worsen with physical exertion or even mild activity. Other signs include the following:

1. Fatigue and breathlessness: Reduced oxygen delivery to tissues makes even everyday tasks feel exhausting.
2. Clubbing of fingers and toes: Chronic low oxygen can cause the fingertips to grow rounder and thicker, leading to a bulbous appearance of the fingertips.
3. Heart palpitations: The heart works harder to compensate for oxygen deprivation.
4. Chest pain: This pain is often a result of strain on the heart or insufficient oxygen.
5. Oedema: There may be swelling in the legs or abdomen due to heart failure.
6. Bleeding tendencies: Patients may bruise easily or experience nosebleeds due to abnormal blood clotting.

The Diagnosis Process

Diagnosing Eisenmenger syndrome typically involves the following steps:

1. Pulse oximetry: A simple test that measures the oxygen levels in the blood
2. Echocardiography: An ultrasound test that checks for structural heart defects and measures blood pressures within the heart
3. CT or MRI scans: Imaging tests used to look closely at the heart and lungs
4. Cardiac catheterisation: A procedure that measures the pressures in the heart and lungs directly

Managing Eisenmenger Syndrome

Although Eisenmenger syndrome cannot be cured, there are various ways to manage the symptoms and improve quality of life.

Treatment Options

1. Oxygen therapy: For some patients, using supplemental oxygen can help alleviate symptoms.
2. Medications:
    a. Pulmonary vasodilators (like bosentan or sildenafil) help lower lung blood pressure.
    b. Anticoagulants prevent blood clots but must be used cautiously.
    c. Diuretics help reduce excess fluid in the body from heart failure.
3. Avoiding triggers: Steering clear of strenuous activities, dehydration or high altitudes can prevent worsening symptoms.
4. Preventing infections: Patients with this condition are particularly vulnerable to infections like infective endocarditis and should seek immediate treatment.

Vaccinations, including those for the flu and pneumonia, are key to prevention.
5. Specialised care: Regular visits with a cardiologist who specialises in congenital heart disease are essential for managing ongoing health.

Living with Eisenmenger Syndrome

An older person living with Eisenmenger syndrome faces both physical and emotional difficulties. Even performing daily activities may require help, and mental health support is significant to address feelings of loneliness or anxiety related to their condition.

While Eisenmenger syndrome is a serious condition, modern treatments and thorough care can enhance both lifespan and quality of life. Recognising symptoms early and getting specialised care can make a considerable difference, reassuring patients and their families.

The Learning

Understanding conditions like Eisenmenger syndrome and other congenital heart diseases helps build awareness about the importance of early detection and intervention. By sharing stories of both victories and struggles, we can educate ourselves and others about the significance of seeking help promptly. This awareness can prepare parents and carers to act quickly when they notice.

> 'Every 5 minutes, 10 children around the world are born with congenital heart disease.'[1]
>
> Children's HeartLink[1]

17

When Emotions Hurt the Heart: Understanding Broken Heart Syndrome

Takotsubo Cardiomyopathy (Broken Heart Syndrome)

Have you ever heard of someone experiencing intense grief or shock and then suddenly feeling chest pain? It might sound like something out of a movie, but in reality, our hearts can react to extreme emotions in surprising ways. Takotsubo cardiomyopathy, commonly known as 'broken heart syndrome', is a temporary heart condition triggered by intense emotional or physical stress. Though it mimics a heart attack, there is no actual blockage in the arteries. Instead, the heart's main pumping chamber temporarily weakens and takes on a balloon-like shape, which affects its ability to pump blood properly.

This condition mostly affects postmenopausal women and is often linked to deeply emotional events such as the loss of a loved one, sudden fear or extreme anxiety. The good news? With proper care, most people recover fully. However, understanding this condition is important because it can sometimes lead to serious complications if not managed correctly. Let us explore this fascinating yet serious heart condition through a real-life case study.

Anjali Sharma

Meet Anjali Sharma, a fifty-six-year-old retired schoolteacher. Generally healthy, she has high blood pressure, which she manages with medication. One evening, Mrs Sharma rushed to the ER with sudden, intense chest pain, shortness of breath and a racing heart. The pain started after she attended the funeral of a close relative – a deeply emotional and stressful event for her.

She described her chest pain as severe, spreading towards her back, but unlike a typical heart attack, she had no nausea or vomiting. For the past week, she had been feeling unusually anxious and stressed, which may have contributed to her symptoms.

Past Medical History

Mrs Sharma had hypertension. It was controlled, and she was taking medicine for that. There was no prior history of CAD, diabetes or dyslipidaemia (abnormal level of fats in blood).

Family History

There was no significant family history of cardiovascular diseases.

Social History

A non-smoker and non-alcoholic, she led a sedentary lifestyle.

Diagnosing the Problem

Step 1: Checking the Heart's Signals

Doctors immediately performed an ECG, which showed changes that looked like a heart attack.

Step 2: Measuring Heart Damage

Blood tests revealed high levels of troponin, a protein released when heart muscles are stressed or damaged. This finding is common in heart attacks, but something was different in Mrs Sharma's case.

Step 3: A Closer Look at the Heart

An echocardiogram showed something unusual – the left ventricle had a balloon-like shape, a classic sign of Takotsubo cardiomyopathy.

Step 4: Checking the Arteries

A coronary angiogram, a test that looks for blockages in the heart's blood vessels, revealed that Mrs Sharma's arteries were clear. This confirmed that she wasn't having a heart attack but rather a case of broken heart syndrome.

Mrs Sharma's Treatment Plan

The First Few Days: Hospital Care

Mrs Sharma was admitted to the hospital for close monitoring. She received oxygen and medications to help her heart recover, including beta-blockers (to calm the heart and reduce stress hormones), ACE inhibitors (to support heart function and reduce strain), blood thinners (to prevent blood clots) and diuretics (to reduce fluid build-up in the lungs).

Healing beyond Medicine: Emotional Support Matters

Since stress was the main trigger, Mrs Sharma also received emotional support. Doctors encouraged her to see a counsellor, practise relaxation techniques like meditation and make time for activities that bring her joy. She was also given dietary counselling for a healthy heart. Since she was leading a sedentary lifestyle, she was encouraged to gradually start physical activity.

The Road to Recovery

One Month Later: A Stronger Heart

Mrs Sharma's symptoms disappeared, and a follow-up heart ultrasound showed her heart function had returned to normal.

Three Months Later: A Healthier Outlook

She continued taking medications and attended counselling sessions. She also adopted a healthier lifestyle by practising stress management, improving her diet and incorporating light exercise.

The Science Behind a Broken Heart

Why Does This Happen?

Takotsubo cardiomyopathy is believed to be caused by a sudden surge of stress hormones, such as adrenaline, which temporarily weakens the heart muscle. The lower part of the heart struggles to contract properly, while the upper part continues working normally, creating the ballooning effect.

What Triggers It?

1. Emotional stress: Grief, heartbreak or major life changes
2. Physical stress: Surgery, infections or accidents
3. Certain medications: Some drugs that stimulate the heart can also trigger it

How Is It Different from a Heart Attack?

Unlike a heart attack, which occurs due to blocked arteries, Takotsubo cardiomyopathy happens because of stress-induced heart muscle weakness. The good news is that it is usually reversible with proper treatment and care.

Are There Any Risks?

Although most people recover completely, some may experience complications like heart failure, irregular heartbeats or blood clots. Hence, early diagnosis and proper treatment are crucial. This condition could reoccur in about 10 per cent to 15 per cent of patients.

The Learning

Mrs Sharma's story highlights a fascinating and important lesson – our hearts and emotions are deeply connected. Takotsubo cardiomyopathy, or broken heart syndrome, shows that extreme emotional stress can physically affect the heart, but with the right care, recovery is possible. Although Takotsubo cardiomyopathy is often reversible, its potential complications necessitate close follow-up and comprehensive care.

While we cannot always avoid stress, we can learn to manage it better. Simple practices like deep breathing, meditation, connectedness with loved ones and professional support when needed can go a long way in keeping our hearts strong and healthy.

At the end of the day, our hearts do more than just pump blood – they also feel. So let us take care of them, both physically and emotionally!

> People with depression or those who are recovering from a heart attack have a lower chance of recovery and a higher risk of death than people without depression.

18

Beyond Snoring: A Scary Wake-Up Call

IMAGINE WAKING UP EVERY morning feeling exhausted, no matter how long you slept. You feel sluggish at work, struggle to concentrate and need multiple cups of coffee just to get through the day. Now, imagine that one day, this exhaustion turns into something much more serious – so serious that you end up in the ER, barely able to stay awake.

This is precisely what happened to a forty-eight-year-old lawyer, Anand Agarwal. A busy professional with long work hours, Anand had been dealing with constant fatigue, loud snoring and weight gain for months. His wife had noticed that he sometimes stopped breathing in his sleep, but he brushed it off, assuming it was nothing serious.

Until one day, it became an emergency.

One morning, Anand's wife noticed something was off. He had been feeling drowsy and confused. He was struggling to stay awake and wasn't responding normally to conversation. When he started having trouble breathing, his wife rushed him to the ER.

At the hospital, doctors found that his body had an extremely high level of carbon dioxide and dangerously low oxygen levels. This meant his lungs weren't removing carbon dioxide properly, leading to a dangerous condition called hypercapnic respiratory failure – a life-threatening state where the body becomes overwhelmed with carbon dioxide and can't get enough oxygen.

The culprit? Severe obstructive sleep apnoea.

What Is Obstructive Sleep Apnoea?

Obstructive sleep apnoea is a common but often under-diagnosed sleep disorder where the airway becomes blocked repeatedly during sleep, causing breathing to stop for short periods. This leads to frequent awakenings throughout the night, poor-quality sleep and low oxygen levels. This sleep disorder is strongly associated with obesity, a sedentary lifestyle and comorbidities such as cardiovascular disease and metabolic syndrome. Severe cases can lead to acute-on-chronic respiratory failure, as in the case of this obese lawyer who presented with altered mental status.

People with this sleep apnoea often:

1. Snore loudly,
2. Feel extremely tired during the day,
3. Experience morning headaches,
4. Struggle with concentration and memory and
5. Have high blood pressure and other health issues.

Case Summary: Understanding the Patient's Condition and Treatment

Medical History

1. Anand had high blood pressure for five years but wasn't taking his medicines regularly.
2. He had type 2 diabetes for three years and was on medication.
3. His daytime sleepiness was affecting his work.

Lifestyle and Risk Factors

1. He had smoked for several years.
2. He did not exercise.
3. He had gained significant weight.
4. He worked long hours, leading to a sedentary lifestyle.

Examination and Tests

At the ER

1. Anand was very drowsy but woke up when spoken to.
2. His oxygen levels were low (88 per cent), and his breathing rate was higher than normal.
3. He was obese (BMI: 36 kg/m^2) with a large neck (45 cm) – both risk factors for sleep apnoea.
4. Snoring and mouth breathing were noticed when he slept in the ER.
5. His mental responses were slow, and he had mild swelling in his legs.

Key Lab and Test Results

1. Blood gas test showed Anand had too much carbon dioxide and too little oxygen in his blood, meaning he wasn't breathing properly.
2. Polysomnography (sleep study that measures how often a person stops breathing during sleep) found that he had severe obstructive sleep apnoea – his breathing stopped or became shallow forty-eight times per hour while sleeping.
3. Heart tests showed mild heart changes due to long-term high blood pressure.
4. Diabetes check showed that his blood sugar was high, indicating poorly controlled diabetes.

This confirmed that his sleep apnoea was not just a minor issue – it was causing serious strain on his body and leading to a dangerous build-up of carbon dioxide in his blood.

Diagnosis

He was diagnosed with severe obstructive sleep apnoea, which had caused respiratory failure by allowing carbon dioxide to build up in his blood. This made him drowsy, confused and extremely tired.

Immediate Treatment in the ER

1. A BiPAP (bilevel positive airway pressure) machine (a type of non-invasive ventilation) was started to help him breathe better. It:
   a. pushed air into his lungs to keep his airways open,
   b. helped clear out excess carbon dioxide and
   c. improved his oxygen levels.
2. Oxygen support was given to keep his oxygen levels above 92 per cent.
3. Monitoring and Adjustments
   a. Doctors closely watched his breathing and mental alertness.
   b. After 4 hours of BiPAP therapy, his condition improved – his carbon dioxide levels dropped, and oxygen levels rose.
4. Other Supportive Measures
   a. The head of his bed was raised to help his breathing.
   b. He was given fluids to keep him hydrated.
   c. Strict BiPAP use was advised to avoid worsening symptoms.

Hospital Stay and Recovery

Anand felt much better within 48 hours of using the BiPAP. Once stable, he was switched to a CPAP (continuous positive airway pressure) machine (similar to BiPAP but for long-term use at home). He was discharged with medications for diabetes and blood pressure.

Long-Term Treatment and Lifestyle Changes

To prevent future complications, he was advised to:

1. use a CPAP machine every night to keep his airways open while sleeping,

2. lose weight through a structured diet and exercise plan,
3. quit smoking to improve his lung function,
4. exercise regularly to help control weight and blood pressure and
5. follow up with a sleep specialist for long-term care.

Obstructive Sleep Apnoea and Its Impact

What Happens and Why Does It Lead to Breathing Problems?

Obstructive sleep apnoea is a condition where a person's airway repeatedly gets blocked during sleep because the muscles in the throat become too relaxed, making it difficult for air to pass through. As a result, the person stops breathing for short periods multiple times throughout the night.

This leads to several problems:

1. Low oxygen levels (hypoxaemia): Since breathing is disrupted, less oxygen reaches the body and brain.
2. High carbon dioxide levels (hypercapnia): When breathing slows or stops, carbon dioxide builds up in the blood instead of being expelled.
3. Inflammation and stress on the body: The repeated drops in oxygen and increase in carbon dioxide create long-term damage, causing inflammation and making the body more sensitive to further breathing issues.

In this case, the patient's obesity played a major role in worsening his condition. Excess fat around his neck made his airway more prone to collapse, and his lung capacity was reduced, making it even harder for him to breathe properly.

Why Is Obstructive Sleep Apnoea Often Diagnosed Late?

Obstructive sleep apnoea is commonly missed because its symptoms seem harmless at first. Many people snore, feel tired during the day or experience occasional sleep disturbances without realising it is a medical condition. This patient ignored symptoms like excessive daytime sleepiness and loud snoring for months, until it became a serious issue.

By the time he came to the hospital, his body had already been struggling for a long time, leading to acute-on-chronic respiratory failure – a dangerous situation where the lungs are unable to remove carbon dioxide effectively. To confirm this sleep disorder, doctors used polysomnography. The patient's test showed severe obstructive sleep apnoea with forty-eight breathing interruptions per hour and a dangerously low oxygen level of 70 per cent while sleeping.

How BiPAP Helps in Emergency Situations

When the patient arrived at the hospital, he was in a critical state – very drowsy, confused and struggling to breathe. Doctors immediately started BiPAP therapy with a special breathing machine that pushes air into the lungs to keep the airway open.

BiPAP helps in three key ways:

1. It improves breathing efficiency. By ensuring enough air reaches the lungs, it lowers carbon dioxide levels in the blood.
2. It increases oxygen levels. More oxygen reaches the brain and other organs, preventing damage.
3. It reduces strain on the lungs and muscles. This helps the patient feel less tired and makes breathing easier.

After just 4 hours of BiPAP therapy, the patient's blood gases showed improvement, meaning his lungs were working better. His oxygen levels increased, and his carbon dioxide levels dropped to a safer range. Over the next two days, he continued to improve significantly.

Long-Term Management: How to Prevent Future Episodes

Obstructive sleep apnoea is not just a short-term problem. If left untreated, it can lead to serious health issues like heart disease, stroke and memory problems. That is why long-term management is essential.

The best treatment for long-term management is CPAP therapy. CPAP provides a steady flow of air to prevent the airway from collapsing during sleep. The patient was discharged with a portable CPAP machine and instructions on how to use it every night.

The Learning

Obstructive sleep apnoea is a serious condition that can cause life-threatening breathing problems if ignored. Obesity significantly increases the risk of this sleep apnoea and worsens breathing difficulties. BiPAP therapy is life-saving for patients in critical condition with high carbon dioxide levels. Long-term CPAP use and lifestyle changes are crucial to prevent future complications. Early diagnosis and treatment can prevent severe respiratory failure and improve quality of life. This case highlights the importance of awareness about obstructive sleep apnoea and its potential dangers. If someone experiences chronic snoring, excessive daytime sleepiness or unexplained fatigue, they should seek medical advice early to avoid serious complications.

> 'Heavy snoring is a risk factor for case fatality and poor short-term prognosis after a first acute myocardial infarction.'
> National Library of Medicine[1]

19

Women and Heart Attacks

Myocardial Infarction in a Twenty-Nine-Year-Old Female

This report tells the story of a twenty-nine-year-old woman who experienced a heart attack, known medically as a myocardial infarction. It highlights how heart attacks in women can differ from those in men. Women often have unique symptoms, risk factors and treatment journeys that are not well understood, making it essential to pay attention to these differences.

Acute myocardial infarction is traditionally considered a condition affecting older males, but its prevalence in younger females is increasing due to lifestyle changes, including smoking, and rising cardiovascular risk factors. Women, especially young ones, often present atypically, leading to delays in diagnosis and treatment. Understanding the gender-based differences in myocardial infarction presentation and outcomes is critical for improving clinical outcomes.

Heart Attacks Aren't Just a Man's Problem

Heart attacks are often thought of as problems that primarily affect older men. However, more young women are experiencing heart attacks, often due to lifestyle choices like smoking and other health risks. Young women tend to show different signs of heart attacks, which can lead to delays in treatment. Recognising these differences is vital to improve care and outcomes for young women experiencing heart attacks.

The Case: A Young Woman in Distress

In our featured case, a twenty-nine-year-old woman went to the ER complaining of sudden chest pain, nausea and trouble breathing. These symptoms had been troubling her for about 3 hours. She described her chest pain as a tight feeling right in the middle of her chest, which also spread to her jaw and back.

Risk Factors: What Affected Her?

- Smoking: She had been smoking about fifteen cigarettes a day for the past ten years.
- Birth control: She had been using oral contraceptives (the pill) for five years.
- Family history: Her father suffered a heart attack at the age of fifty-five.
- No major health issues: She had not been diagnosed with high blood pressure, diabetes or any other significant health problems.

Examination: What the Doctors Found

When the woman arrived at the ER, the medical team observed her vital signs. Her blood pressure was 130/85 mmHg and heart rate was 102 beats per minute, which was a bit fast. Oxygen levels were 97 per cent on room air, which was acceptable. During the examination, the doctors noted that she was sweating a bit and appeared anxious.

Investigations: Understanding What Happened

To learn more about her condition, the medical team conducted several tests:

1. ECG: This test showed changes in certain areas of her heart, indicating a heart attack affecting the lower part of the heart.
2. Cardiac biomarkers: A blood test showed an elevated level of a protein (troponin) that indicates heart damage.

3. Echocardiography: An ultrasound of the heart showed some reduced movement in the lower wall of the heart but good overall heart function.
4. Coronary angiography: This procedure showed a blockage in one of the main arteries.

Management: Steps to Help Her Recover
1. Immediate treatment: They gave her medications, including aspirin, clopidogrel and atorvastatin, right away. They also performed a procedure called primary percutaneous coronary intervention, which opened the blocked artery.
2. Medications after the procedure: After the procedure, she received additional medications to prevent future clots and manage her heart.
3. Lifestyle changes: The doctors discussed the importance of quitting smoking and the potential risks of the birth control pills she was using.

Understanding the Differences in Heart Attacks between Men and Women

How Symptoms Differ

Men typically experience strong chest pain, often described as pressure or a squeezing feeling, and may feel sweaty and generally uncomfortable.

Women are more likely to experience unusual signs like nausea, feeling faint, extreme fatigue and shortness of breath. When women do have chest pain, it is usually milder and may be described as tightness rather than pain. This woman's symptoms fit the pattern often seen in females.

Different Risk Factors

Men

Often, risk factors include lifestyle habits like smoking, high blood pressure, high cholesterol and diabetes.

Women

Women have certain unique risk factors for heart problems due to hormonal changes. For example, using birth control pills (oral contraceptives) can affect blood flow and clotting. Complications during pregnancy, such as pre-eclampsia (high blood pressure) or GDM (high blood sugar levels during pregnancy), can also increase the risk of heart disease later in life.

Smoking and birth control pills are a dangerous combination. When women smoke while taking birth control pills, their risk of having a heart attack increases significantly. Both smoking and birth control pills make the blood more likely to clot. These clots can block blood flow to the heart, leading to a heart attack, especially in younger women.

Autoimmune diseases also affect the heart. Women are more likely than men to have autoimmune diseases like lupus or rheumatoid arthritis. These conditions cause chronic inflammation, which can damage blood vessels over time and increase the risk of heart disease. Inflammation makes arteries more likely to develop blockages, leading to serious heart problems.

In this specific case, the woman was both a smoker and a user of oral contraceptives. This combination likely played a major role in triggering her acute thrombotic event (a sudden, serious blood clot that can block arteries and cause a heart attack or stroke). Her lifestyle choices, combined with the natural risk factors women face, significantly increased her chances of experiencing this life-threatening condition.

Causes of Heart Attacks

Men often suffer from a condition called atherosclerosis, which involves fatty deposits blocking blood vessels.

In women, younger females can experience other issues like spasms in their blood vessels or conditions that affect blood flow, and these differences can complicate their treatment.

Understanding the Pathophysiology of Heart Disease in Men and Women

Men

Atherosclerosis, the build-up of fatty deposits (plaques) in the arteries over time, is the primary cause of heart attacks and other serious heart problems in men. The biggest danger comes when one of these plaques ruptures (breaks open). When this happens, the body sees it as an injury and tries to form a blood clot (thrombosis) to heal it. If the clot becomes too large, it can completely block the artery (vessel occlusion), stopping blood flow to the heart and causing a heart attack.

Women

In younger women, heart problems are often caused by factors other than atherosclerosis:

1. Coronary artery spasm is a temporary tightening of the arteries, which can block blood flow to the heart even if there are no plaques.
2. Spontaneous coronary artery dissection is a rare condition where the inner layers of an artery tear, leading to a blockage.
3. Microvascular dysfunction is a problem with the tiny blood vessels in the heart, where they don't expand properly, reducing blood supply even if the main arteries are clear.
4. Inflammation and hormones also affect women's heart health more than men's. Oestrogen and other hormones influence how blood vessels work (endothelial function) and how arteries react to different stressors (coronary reactivity).
5. Autoimmune diseases, which are more common in women, cause chronic inflammation that can make arteries more vulnerable.

The patient's angiography did not show any significant atherosclerosis, meaning she did not have major plaque build-up blocking her arteries. Instead, her heart event was likely caused by a sudden blood clot (thrombotic event). Her smoking and use of oral contraceptives likely played a major role in triggering the event.

Challenges in Diagnosis

Women often don't receive quick treatment because their symptoms can be misattributed to non-cardiac causes, such as stress or gastrointestinal issues. Hence, care that could prevent serious complications is often delayed. In this case, the woman's age and gender could have led to potential misunderstandings about her symptoms if it weren't for the clear signs shown on her ECG.

Younger women who experience a myocardial infarction (heart attack) are often misdiagnosed because their symptoms can be atypical compared to the classic 'crushing chest pain' commonly seen in men. Instead of severe chest pain, women – especially younger ones – may present with symptoms such as neck, jaw or back pain (which can be mistaken for musculoskeletal issues); shortness of breath, dizziness or fatigue (which may be attributed to anxiety or panic attacks) and nausea or indigestion (which can be misdiagnosed as a gastrointestinal issue). Since heart attacks are more commonly associated with older men, doctors may not immediately suspect one in a younger woman, increasing the risk of misdiagnosis.

Disparities in Treatment

Men typically receive more aggressive interventions such as procedures to open blocked arteries or bypass surgeries.

Women may face barriers in accessing these same treatments. Healthcare providers might not prescribe necessary medications as readily to women. Additionally, women can experience social factors that complicate their healthcare, like caregiving responsibilities and financial constraints, further limiting their access to the care they need. Thankfully, in this case, prompt intervention with percutaneous coronary intervention was critical for the woman's recovery.

Prognosis and Outcomes

Men generally fare better in terms of immediate recovery due to earlier identification and treatment of their heart issues.

Women often face higher rates of complications during hospitalisation, such as heart failure, shock and arrhythmias, and poorer long-term outcomes. Factors contributing to these disparities include misdiagnosis, insufficient treatment and a lack of aggressive management for their health risks. While younger women may recover better than older women, they still have a heightened risk of facing heart-related issues later if their risk factors – like smoking – are not addressed.

Addressing the Challenges of Heart Attacks in Young Women

This case emphasises how challenging it can be to recognise and manage heart attacks in young women. It highlights the importance of understanding the different symptoms, risk factors and care needs specific to women to enhance their health outcomes.

Key Points for Addressing Heart Attacks in Young Women

1. Educate everyone: Healthcare providers and women themselves should be better informed about the unusual ways heart attacks can show up in women.
2. Control risk factors: Strong measures must be taken against modifiable risk factors, like quitting smoking and discussing safe alternatives to hormonal contraceptives, which can pose additional risks.
3. Timely diagnosis: Rapid assessment using ECGs and other tests is crucial for women with atypical symptoms.

Recognising signs early can save lives.
4. Post-heart attack support: After a heart attack, women should receive comprehensive rehabilitation and mental health support. They are more susceptible to feelings of anxiety or depression during recovery.

The Learning

This case showcases the complex nature of heart attacks in a young female smoker and underscores the influence of lifestyle and hormonal factors on cardiovascular health. Differences in how men and women experience and respond to heart attacks emphasise the necessity for a customised approach to heart health. If these disparities are acknowledged and actively addressed, healthcare providers can enhance the quality of care for women experiencing heart attacks, ultimately reducing long-term cardiovascular risks.

> 'Cardiovascular disease is responsible for 30 per cent of deaths in women each year – over twice as many deaths in women each year as all forms of cancer combined.'
> World Heart Federation[1]

20

Right Heart Failure in Alcoholic Liver Disease

A Complex Medical Challenge

When the liver is damaged, it can cause high blood pressure in the portal vein (the vein that carries blood from the intestines to the liver), which results in increased blood flow back to the right side of the heart, leading to chronic volume overload. Severe tricuspid regurgitation (TR) occurs because of the following reasons:

1. Valve stretching: The area around the tricuspid valve becomes enlarged, making it less effective.
2. Right ventricle dysfunction: The right ventricle can't pump blood forward efficiently, worsening TR.
3. Congested liver: Blood flow gets backed up in the liver, contributing to more pressure on the heart and further impairing its function.

Understanding the Progression of TR

As TR worsens, it leads to a damaging cycle: the heart gets overloaded with volume, fluid builds up in the body and blood flow to the liver decreases. This makes liver health even worse and complicates the ability to qualify for a transplant.

Clinical Presentation: Recognising Symptoms of Right Heart Failure

Symptoms of Right Heart Failure

1. Feeling tired and weak: This happens because the heart is not pumping enough blood.

2. Swelling in the body: Extra fluid in the body leads to swelling, particularly in the legs and feet.
3. Fluid in the abdomen: Excess fluid build-up can cause discomfort in the abdomen due to pressure from portal hypertension.
4. Visible swelling in neck veins: Enlarged veins in the neck show the heart is under pressure.

Signs of Severe TR

1. Holosystolic murmur, a specific heart sound: A continuous sound (murmur) can be heard, especially when taking a deep breath.
2. Liver issues: Common issues are an enlarged liver (hepatomegaly), fluid build-up in the abdomen (ascites) and a pulsing liver, all due to high blood pressure in veins.

Diagnostic Evaluation

Echocardiography

1. Severity of TR: This condition means that the tricuspid valve (which separates the right atrium or the right upper chamber and right ventricle or the right lower chamber) is leaking blood backwards. It is classified as mild, moderate or severe, depending on how much blood is leaking and how wide the jet of backward blood flow appears on the ultrasound.
2. Tricuspid annular dilation (more than 40 mm in the apical four-chamber view): The tricuspid annulus is the ring-like structure where the tricuspid valve is attached. If this ring stretches beyond 40 mm, it suggests that the valve is enlarging, which can worsen leakage.
3. Right ventricular function: The right ventricle is responsible for pumping blood to the lungs. This test checks the size of the right ventricle (enlarged or normal), the pressure in that ventricle, which indicates if there is strain on the heart, and the strain (deformation)

of the right ventricle muscle, which shows how well it contracts.

Liver Function Tests and Imaging

These tests check if the heart problem is affecting the liver. They check the severity of hepatic dysfunction and portal hypertension. When the heart doesn't pump blood properly, blood can back up into the liver, leading to swelling and liver damage. Portal hypertension means increased pressure in the liver's blood vessels, which can cause complications like fluid build-up in the abdomen.

The tests also exclude hepatocellular carcinoma (liver cancer) or other complications. Since liver disease can lead to cancer or other serious conditions, imaging (like ultrasound or CT scan) is done to rule out these issues.

Cardiac MRI

A cardiac MRI is a detailed scan of the heart using magnetic fields and radio waves. It provides a more accurate measurement of right ventricle size and function than an echocardiogram, especially if the ultrasound images are unclear. This is useful in cases where the heart is enlarged or there are doubts about the severity of the problem.

Haemodynamic Assessment (Checking Blood Flow and Pressures in the Heart)

Right heart catheterisation is a procedure where a thin tube (catheter) is inserted into a vein and guided into the right side of the heart. It directly measures the pressure in the heart and lungs, helping doctors determine how well the heart is pumping blood, if the patient has pulmonary hypertension (high blood pressure in the lungs) and whether this hypertension is due to a heart problem (post-capillary) or another issue (pre-capillary).

This evaluation helps doctors understand the severity of the condition and decide on the best treatment.

Challenges in Management

Managing severe TR in someone who also has liver disease and is waiting for a liver transplant is very complicated because both the heart and liver are affected. Here's why.

High Surgical Risk

The heart and liver are both weak, making any major surgery dangerous. If the patient undergoes open-heart surgery to replace the tricuspid valve, they face a higher chance of complications, such as severe bleeding (because liver disease affects blood clotting) and infections (because liver disease weakens immunity and healing).

Volume Overload

TR causes fluid to back up into the body, leading to swelling (oedema), fluid in the lungs and congestion in organs like the liver and kidneys. Doctors try to fix this using diuretics (water pills) to remove excess fluid.

However, the challenge is that if too much fluid is removed, it can reduce blood flow to the kidneys, making kidney function worse — especially in patients with hepatorenal syndrome (a condition where liver failure leads to kidney failure).

Pulmonary Hypertension

Pulmonary hypertension means high blood pressure in the lungs, which makes it harder for the heart to pump blood. TR causes blood to back up into the lungs, increasing lung pressure. Portal hypertension (high pressure in the liver's blood vessels) can also contribute to pulmonary hypertension. This combination makes both medical treatment and surgery more difficult as it increases the risk of heart and lung failure.

Timing of Intervention

Doctors must carefully plan when to fix the heart valve because doing it too early or too late can be dangerous. If the valve surgery is done too soon, the patient may not be eligible for a liver transplant due to surgical risks. If the valve surgery is delayed too long, the heart may become too weak to support a successful liver transplant. Doctors must coordinate the heart and liver treatments to ensure the best possible outcome for both organs.

Therapeutic Approaches

Medical Management

Even though medical treatment doesn't directly fix TR, it can help ease symptoms and prepare patients for further treatments.

1. Diuretics are medications that help eliminate excess fluid but must be used carefully to avoid harming the kidneys. Doctors often combine different types of diuretics to enhance effectiveness.
2. Pulmonary vasodilators like sildenafil or macitentan may help lower blood pressure in the lungs, but they are used selectively.
3. Inotropic support, additional support to help the heart pump more effectively, might be necessary for those with weakened right ventricle function.

Interventional Strategies: Options for Repairing the Heart

Tricuspid Valve Replacement

1. When it is needed: This surgery is considered when TR is severe and symptoms persist despite medical treatment or when right ventricle function is significantly impaired, making it tough to qualify for transplant.
2. Challenges: Surgery carries high risks for those with serious liver disease and can lead to complications with the artificial valve, such as blood clots or infections.
3. Timing considerations: Often, this procedure is postponed until the liver transplant is done, unless the severe TR is a barrier to being eligible for the transplant.

TriClip Procedure

The TriClip is a minimally invasive treatment option designed to repair the tricuspid valve without the need for major surgery. It is a small device placed inside the heart using a catheter without open surgery to help reduce the valve leak.

1. Advantages: This method reduces TR effectively while lowering the risk of complications that come with open-heart surgery.
2. Selecting patients: It is ideal for patients who have high surgical risks but whose right ventricular function is still acceptable. A thorough assessment of the heart's structure and function is crucial before continuing with this procedure.
3. Evidence of effectiveness: Studies show that using the TriClip has successfully improved patients' capacity to function and provided relief from symptoms in individuals at high risk.

Liver Transplantation: Addressing the Root Cause

The primary goal of liver transplant surgery is to treat the underlying causes of congestive hepatopathy and liver cirrhosis, often leading to improved TR and right ventricular function.

1. Benefits of liver transplant: A transplant can dramatically enhance survival rates and improve quality of life for patients suffering from these conditions.
2. Pre-transplant preparation: It is important to address significant TR before performing a transplant in carefully chosen patients to improve overall outcomes.
3. Post-transplant considerations: After the transplant, patients usually see improvement in right ventricular function and TR due to reduced blood pressure in the veins and less strain on the liver.

Combined Heart and Liver Transplantation: A Rare Need

In some special cases, patients might need both heart and liver transplants at the same time, though this is only performed at select medical centres and requires careful consideration of the risks involved.

Case-Based Considerations

Who Is the Patient?

The patient is a fifty-eight-year-old man with alcohol-related liver disease. His MELD (Model for End-stage Liver Disease) score is 18, meaning he has moderate to severe liver disease and is waiting for a liver transplant. There is severe TR. His heart's tricuspid valve is leaking badly. His right heart chamber is enlarged and not pumping well. His liver disease has caused high pressure in the liver's blood vessels, leading to fluid build-up in the belly (ascites) that does not improve with usual treatments.

How Should This Patient Be Managed?

Optimise Medical Therapy (Start with Medications and Monitoring)

1. Use diuretics carefully to remove extra fluid from the body. Check kidney function regularly since removing too much fluid can harm the kidneys.
2. Consider using low-dose pulmonary vasodilators (special medications that relax blood vessels in the lungs) if lung pressure is high, making it easier for the heart to pump blood.

Evaluate for TriClip

TriClip may improve blood circulation, stabilise the patient's condition and increase the chances of a successful liver transplant.

Coordinate Multidisciplinary Care (Team Approach to Treatment)

The heart, liver and transplant teams must work together to decide the best timing for any treatment to ensure that heart treatments don't interfere with the liver transplant process.

Proceed with Liver Transplantation When Possible

Once the patient is stable enough, doctors will move forward with liver transplantation. The patient's heart function needs to be closely monitored to ensure it recovers well after the transplant.

Prognosis

If No Treatment Is Given (Worst-Case Scenario)

The heart will pump less efficiently, leading to right heart failure. The body will retain more fluid, worsening swelling, breathing problems and liver damage. The patient may become too sick for a liver transplant, meaning they lose their chance for a life-saving procedure.

If Treatment Is Given on Time

Procedures like TriClip can stabilise the patient, reduce heart strain and improve blood flow. This increases the chances of a successful liver transplant and a better long-term outcome.

What Happens After a Successful Liver Transplant?

The heart may recover on its own. In many cases, fixing the liver also helps the heart work better, especially if lung pressure decreases after the transplant. If needed, additional heart treatments can be done after the liver is stable.

The Learning

Managing right heart failure with severe TR in alcoholic liver disease requires a comprehensive, patient-centred approach. Interventions like the TriClip procedure offer hope for bridging patients to liver transplantation, minimising surgical risks while improving symptoms. Collaborative care among cardiologists, hepatologists and transplant teams is crucial for optimising outcomes. By addressing both cardiac and hepatic components of this complex condition, patients can achieve a better quality of life and improved survival prospects.

> 'When it comes to heart disease, the number one thing that comes to mind is smoking, and we do not think about alcohol as one of the vital signs. I think a lot more awareness is needed, and alcohol should be part of routine health assessments moving forward.'
> Jamal Rana, MD, PhD, FACC, a cardiologist with The Permanente Medical Group[1]

21

A Pregnancy Complicated by Rheumatic Heart Disease

PREGNANCY IS A BEAUTIFUL journey, but it can become challenging for women with certain medical conditions, especially heart diseases. One such condition is rheumatic heart disease (RHD), which can make pregnancy a high-risk situation. Let me share the story of one of my patients – a twenty-eight-year-old woman named Meera – who successfully navigated pregnancy with RHD.

Meera's Background

Meera came to my clinic in her first trimester of pregnancy, accompanied by her husband. She had been experiencing fatigue, breathlessness and occasional palpitations. Her symptoms started worsening as her pregnancy progressed, especially when climbing stairs or doing light chores. She had been diagnosed with rheumatic fever as a child but hadn't followed up for years.

Understanding RHD

RHD is a long-term complication of rheumatic fever, which is caused by an untreated streptococcal throat infection, a sore throat caused by the *Streptococcus* bacteria (commonly known as 'strep throat') that is not treated with antibiotics. In simple terms, the infection triggers the body's immune system to attack the heart valves, leading to damage and scarring. This damage makes it harder for the valves to open and close properly, affecting blood flow through the heart.

The most commonly affected valve is the mitral valve (one of the four valves in the heart), which may either be narrow (mitral stenosis), making it harder for blood to flow from the left atrium to the left ventricle, or leak (mitral regurgitation [MR]), allowing blood to flow backwards into the atrium.

In Meera's case, she had severe mitral stenosis, which had gone undiagnosed until her pregnancy brought it to light.

How Pregnancy Affects the Heart

During pregnancy, a woman's heart works harder than usual. Blood volume increases by about 30 to 50 per cent to support the growing baby. The heart rate also rises, and these changes put extra stress on a damaged heart. For someone with RHD, this can worsen symptoms such as shortness of breath, swelling in the legs, fatigue and palpitations. For Meera, her symptoms were a result of her heart struggling to pump enough blood through the narrowed mitral valve.

Risks and Complications

Managing RHD in pregnancy requires balancing the health of the mother and the baby. The risks include the following:

- Heart failure: The heart already works harder during pregnancy. If the heart is weak or damaged (as in RHD), it may struggle to pump enough blood.
- Blood clots: Poor blood flow through a damaged valve increases the risk of clots, which can cause strokes or complications in pregnancy.
- Arrhythmias: Irregular heartbeats may develop due to the strain on the heart.
- Delivery risks: Labour and delivery further stress the heart, requiring careful planning.

Diagnosis

To confirm Meera's condition, we performed these tests:

1. Echocardiography (2D echo) showed severe narrowing of the mitral valve (stenosis) with a valve area of 1.0 cm^2 (normal is 4–6 cm^2). Blood was struggling to flow through the narrowed valve, causing increased pressure in her lungs.
2. Chest X-ray revealed an enlarged heart and signs of congestion in her lungs.
3. ECG showed AFib, an irregular heartbeat commonly seen in RHD patients with mitral stenosis.
4. Blood tests helped check for anaemia, which can worsen symptoms of RHD.

Treatment and Management

Managing RHD in pregnancy requires a multidisciplinary approach involving a cardiologist, obstetrician and, sometimes, a cardiac surgeon. Here's how we managed Meera's case:

Medication

We gave Meera three types of medicines to help her heart work better:

1. Beta-blockers (like metoprolol) to control her heart rate and reduce the workload on her heart
2. Diuretics (like furosemide) to reduce fluid build-up in her lungs, relieving breathlessness
3. Anticoagulants (like low molecular weight heparin) to prevent blood clots, especially since pregnancy increases the risk of clotting

Lifestyle Adjustments

To make sure her heart didn't get too stressed, we advised some lifestyle changes. Meera was advised to avoid strenuous activities and take frequent breaks to reduce her heart's workload. We also recommended a low-salt diet to prevent fluid retention and a balanced diet for her and the baby's nutrition.

Regular Monitoring

Because Meera's condition was serious, she needed frequent check-ups to monitor her heart function and ensure her baby was growing well. We performed periodic echocardiograms to assess her valve function and lung pressures.

A Critical Decision: Balloon Valvuloplasty

Around the twenty-fourth week of pregnancy, Meera's symptoms worsened significantly. Her breathlessness became severe, and she started experiencing fainting episodes. We decided to perform a percutaneous balloon mitral valvuloplasty – a minimally invasive procedure to open the narrowed mitral valve.

In this procedure, a catheter with a balloon was inserted through a vein in her leg and guided to her mitral valve. The balloon was inflated to widen the valve, improving blood flow.

The procedure was successful, and Meera's symptoms improved dramatically. Her heart could now pump blood more efficiently, reducing the strain on her and her baby.

Planning Delivery

Ensuring a safe delivery was a top priority, given the added risks associated with the heart condition. A well-coordinated plan was put in place to minimise complications and support both mother and baby.

1. Vaginal delivery was preferred as it is generally safer than a caesarean section for heart patients.
2. Labour was carefully monitored with a team of specialists ready to manage any complications.

The Delivery

At 37 weeks, Meera went into labour. She was admitted to the hospital, where a team of cardiologists, obstetricians and anaesthetists closely monitored her. The labour was smooth, and she gave birth to a healthy baby boy.

After delivery, Meera's heart was under extra stress as her blood volume rapidly shifted. She was closely monitored in the ICU for 48 hours to ensure her heart remained stable.

Postpartum Care

RHD doesn't end with delivery – it requires lifelong management. After delivery, we focused on the following:

1. Continuation of medications: Meera stayed on anticoagulants for a few months to prevent postpartum blood clots.
2. Follow-up: She underwent regular check-ups to monitor her valve function and prevent further damage.
3. Family planning: We discussed the importance of consulting a cardiologist before planning future pregnancies. Meera was advised to consider valve repair or replacement if her symptoms worsened.

The Learning

1. Early diagnosis is key: Meera's story highlights the importance of early detection of RHD. Regular check-ups after rheumatic fever can prevent long-term complications.
2. Multidisciplinary care: Managing RHD in pregnancy requires a team approach. Coordination between cardiology and obstetrics was crucial for Meera's successful outcome.
3. Awareness: Many women with RHD don't realise they have a heart condition until pregnancy exacerbates the

symptoms. Public awareness about rheumatic fever and its link to RHD is essential.
4. Modern treatments: Procedures like balloon valvuloplasty can significantly improve outcomes for pregnant women with RHD.

A Message to Women with RHD

If you have RHD and are planning a pregnancy, remember:

1. Consult your cardiologist early to assess your heart's condition.
2. Pregnancy is possible, but it requires careful planning and monitoring.
3. Advances in medicine and minimally invasive procedures have made it safer than ever to manage RHD during pregnancy.

Meera's journey was challenging, but with timely intervention and expert care, both she and her baby emerged healthy and strong. Her story highlights the courage of a mother and the remarkable advances in modern medicine.

> Heart disease can be silent for years. Diabetics, women and older adults may not feel chest pain even with severe heart disease.

22

A Second Chance: Treating Heart Failure and Severe Mitral Regurgitation with MitraClip

MEET MRS VERMA, AN eighty-two-year-old grandmother who had always been the heart of her family. However, her health began to decline. She struggled with severe shortness of breath, swollen legs and profound fatigue. Even simple activities like walking to the bathroom left her gasping for air. Her doctors diagnosed her with congestive heart failure caused by severe MR – a serious condition where the mitral valve in her heart leaked blood backwards instead of pumping it forwards. At her age, traditional open-heart surgery was too risky. Thankfully, a revolutionary procedure called MitraClip offered her a second chance at life.

What Is MR?

The mitral valve is one of four valves in the heart, located between the left atrium and the left ventricle. It works like a one-way door, allowing blood to flow forwards while preventing backflow.

In MR, the valve becomes faulty and allows blood to leak backwards into the left atrium when the heart contracts. Over time, this forces the heart to work harder, leading to symptoms of congestive heart failure such as:

1. severe shortness of breath, especially when lying down or during physical activity;

2. fatigue and inability to perform daily activities;
3. swollen feet, ankles or abdomen (fluid retention) and
4. persistent cough, often with frothy sputum.

Causes of MR

1. Degenerative valve disease: Age-related wear and tear on the valve
2. Functional MR: Caused by an enlarged heart due to conditions like heart failure or a previous heart attack

For Mrs Verma, the cause of degenerative MR was ageing.

Mrs Verma's Story: From Symptoms to Diagnosis

Mrs Verma had first noticed her symptoms a year earlier. Initially, she thought her breathlessness was just part of getting older. But as her condition worsened, she couldn't even lie flat without feeling like she was suffocating. Her family noticed she looked tired all the time and had swollen legs.

Her doctor performed a physical examination, during which he detected a heart murmur. This led to an echocardiogram, which revealed the following:

1. Severe MR, with over half of the blood leaking backwards into her left atrium
2. An enlarged left atrium and left ventricle, signs of a heart struggling to cope
3. Congestive heart failure, a chronic condition in which the heart fails to pump enough blood to meet the body's requirements

Mrs Verma was referred to a cardiologist specialising in valve diseases. They explained that her heart was under severe strain, and without treatment, her condition would continue to worsen.

Why Surgery Wasn't an Option

The standard treatment for severe MR is open-heart surgery to repair or replace the mitral valve. However, Mrs Verma's age and frail health made surgery extremely risky. Her other medical conditions, including borderline kidney function and mild lung disease, added to the risks. This is a common dilemma for older patients with severe MR. Fortunately, there's a minimally invasive alternative: MitraClip.

What Is MitraClip?

The MitraClip procedure involves attaching a small clip to the mitral valve to reduce the backward flow of blood. It is performed using a catheter-based approach, which avoids the need for open-heart surgery.

Here's how it works:

1. Accessing the heart: A small incision is made in the groin, and a catheter is inserted into a large vein. The catheter is guided to the heart using X-ray and ultrasound imaging.
2. Positioning the clip: The MitraClip device is carefully positioned over the leaking part of the mitral valve.
3. Securing the valve: The clip is attached to the valve, pulling the two leaky flaps closer together and reducing the backward flow of blood.
4. Immediate improvement: Blood flow improves immediately, and the heart no longer has to work as hard.

The entire procedure takes about 1–2 hours, and most patients are discharged within 1–3 days.

Mrs Verma's MitraClip Journey

Before the procedure, Mrs Verma underwent a series of tests to confirm that she was a good candidate for MitraClip, including:

1. transoesophageal echocardiography, a detailed ultrasound of the heart done by passing a probe down your oesophagus, giving a clearer view, especially useful before surgery to assess the valve structure, and
2. A CT scan to map the heart and blood vessels.

Her cardiology team explained the procedure, and Mrs Verma was reassured that she would be sedated but not fully unconscious during the procedure.

The MitraClip Procedure

On the Day of the Procedure

Mrs Verma was prepared and ready for treatment.

Steps Taken During the MitraClip Procedure
1. A catheter was inserted through a vein in her groin and guided to her heart.
2. Using advanced imaging techniques, the cardiologist positioned the MitraClip precisely on her mitral valve.
3. Upon reaching the correct placement, the clip was deployed, which effectively reduced the leakage of blood to a less severe level.

Mrs Verma remained stable throughout the procedure, and there were no complications.

Recovery and Results

Within hours of the procedure, Mrs Verma noticed a dramatic difference. She could breathe comfortably while lying flat for the first time in months.

Over the Next Few Days
1. Her energy levels improved significantly, and she found herself feeling less fatigued.

2. The swelling in her legs began to decrease, indicating her body was responding positively to the treatment.
3. Mrs Verma was discharged from the hospital just 48 hours after her procedure, which is a testament to the effectiveness of MitraClip.

By her first follow-up appointment, Mrs Verma had returned to enjoying light household activities and cherishing time spent with her family, a clear indication of her enhanced quality of life.

Benefits of MitraClip

MitraClip offers several key advantages, especially for older patients facing severe MR:

1. Minimal invasiveness: The procedure does not require open-heart surgery or large incisions, allowing for safer treatment with less trauma to the body.
2. Quick recovery: Most patients can return home within just a few days compared to longer hospital stays for traditional surgeries.
3. Improved quality of life: Many experience significant relief from debilitating symptoms such as shortness of breath and extreme fatigue, allowing them to engage more fully in daily life.
4. Reduced hospitalisations: Research indicates that patients receiving the MitraClip procedure have fewer readmissions for heart failure, suggesting better overall heart health management after treatment.

Several concerns and myths exist regarding the MitraClip procedure, which are important to address:

Is It as Effective as Surgery?

MitraClip has been shown to provide substantial symptom relief and improve survival rates for patients who are not candidates for surgical interventions.

Am I Too Old for the Procedure?

The MitraClip procedure is specifically designed to be safe for older and high-risk patients, meaning that age should not deter anyone from seeking this treatment option.

Will the Clip Last Long?

Research indicates that the MitraClip remains effective over multiple years for most patients, providing long-term relief from symptoms.

What Makes MitraClip a Game Changer?

Severe MR was once considered untreatable in many older or high-risk patients. MitraClip has changed that by offering a safe and effective option with minimal risks. For patients like Mrs Verma, it means living a fuller, healthier life without the burden of heart failure symptoms.

Take-Home Message

The story of Mrs Verma serves as a powerful reminder that age should not prevent individuals from receiving vital medical treatments. No one should have to endure the debilitating effects of heart failure due to severe MR. If you or someone you love has received this diagnosis, it is essential to consult with a healthcare provider about all available treatment options, including the MitraClip procedure. Early diagnosis and treatment can significantly improve quality of life and provide much-needed relief.

Heart disease is a major cause of disability that can limit activity and erode quality of life for older people. Talk with a doctor if you have any concerns about your heart as you age.

23

Life 2.0: How a Seventy-Six-Year-Old Beat Heart Trouble with a Simple Procedure

MEET MR SHARMA, a seventy-six-year-old retired teacher, lifelong smoker and someone living with chronic obstructive pulmonary disease. For years, he ignored symptoms like breathlessness, fatigue and chest discomfort, attributing them to his age and smoking history. However, what seemed like 'normal ageing' masked a serious heart condition – severe aortic stenosis, a life-threatening problem that is often missed in its early stages. Thanks to modern medicine and a minimally invasive procedure called transcatheter aortic valve replacement (TAVR), Mr Sharma has been given a new lease on life.

What Is Aortic Stenosis?

The aortic valve is one of the heart's main valves, acting like a door that allows blood to flow from the heart into the aorta and then to the rest of the body. In aortic stenosis, this valve becomes stiff and narrowed, making it harder for blood to flow. Think of it as a rusty door that doesn't open properly.

Over time, the heart has to work harder to push blood through the narrow valve, leading to symptoms like:

1. shortness of breath;
2. chest pain or tightness (angina);
3. fatigue, especially during physical activities;

4. dizziness or fainting spells and
5. swollen feet or ankles (a sign of heart failure in advanced cases).

How Did Mr Sharma's Aortic Stenosis Go Unnoticed?

Initially, Mr Sharma's symptoms were subtle. As a smoker with chronic obstructive pulmonary disease, he was used to shortness of breath and fatigue, and so was his doctor. For years, these symptoms were chalked up to lung disease with little thought given to his heart. This is a common story as early signs of aortic stenosis often overlap with other conditions like chronic obstructive pulmonary disease, making it easy to miss.

It wasn't until Mr Sharma fainted while walking to the market that doctors decided to dig deeper. A thorough physical examination revealed a heart murmur – an abnormal sound caused by turbulent blood flow through the narrowed valve. This prompted an echocardiogram (echo), which confirmed the diagnosis of severe aortic stenosis.

What Makes Severe Aortic Stenosis So Dangerous?

Severe aortic stenosis can be extremely dangerous and is often considered a silent killer. Without treatment, it can lead to severe complications:

1. Heart failure, where the heart can no longer pump blood efficiently
2. Irregular heartbeats that could potentially result in sudden death
3. Stroke, which can occur if blood clots form due to slowed blood flow and travel to the brain

Once the symptoms arise, the average remaining life expectancy without treatment drops to just two to three years.

Treatment Options: Surgery versus TAVR

Traditionally, this condition was treated with open-heart surgery, where the damaged valve is replaced with an artificial one. However, this is a major operation that carries significant risks, especially for elderly patients like Mr Sharma with other health issues such as chronic obstructive pulmonary disease.

Enter TAVR, a game-changing, minimally invasive procedure.

What Is TAVR and How Does It Work?

TAVR (also called transcatheter aortic valve implantation) involves replacing the damaged valve without open-heart surgery. Instead, a new valve is inserted through a catheter placed in an artery, usually in the groin.

Here's how it works:

1. Gaining access to the artery: A small cut is made in the groin area, and a catheter (tube) is guided up to the heart.
2. Positioning the new valve: The replacement valve, made from a combination of metal and animal tissue, is inserted into the old, narrowed valve.
3. Deploying the valve: The new valve expands either by using a balloon or through its own self-expanding mechanism, pushing the old valve aside.

The entire TAVR process generally takes about 1 to 2 hours, with most patients remaining awake but sedated throughout the procedure, which reduces the need for the risks associated with general anaesthesia.

Why TAVR Was the Perfect Solution for Mr Sharma

For Mr Sharma, traditional open-heart surgery wasn't an option due to his age and underlying respiratory issues. TAVR provided multiple advantages tailored to his needs:

1. Minimal invasiveness: Unlike open-heart surgery, TAVR doesn't require the chest to be opened or the use of a heart-lung machine, making it a less complicated procedure.
2. Quicker recovery: Most patients can return home within two to three days after TAVR, whereas those who undergo open-heart surgery may need several weeks to recover.
3. Lower risk of complications: This aspect is especially crucial for high-risk patients like Mr Sharma.

Mr Sharma's Journey to Recovery

After his diagnosis, Mr Sharma was referred to a cardiology team specialising in structural heart diseases. They assessed his case and determined he was a good candidate for TAVR.

Before the Procedure

Mr Sharma underwent a CT angiogram to visualise his arteries, ensuring that the new valve could be safely delivered. His heart and lung functions were enhanced through medication, and he was educated regarding the procedure and what to expect during recovery.

The Day of the TAVR Procedure

The medical team made an incision to insert a catheter through his femoral artery in the groin. With the help of real-time X-ray imaging, they skilfully guided the new valve to the correct position in his heart. The replacement valve was deployed successfully, restoring blood flow through the aortic valve immediately. The entire procedure lasted only 90 minutes, and importantly, Mr Sharma experienced no complications.

Recovery and Remarkable Results

After the procedure, Mr Sharma spent some time under observation overnight in the ICU and was discharged just 48 hours later. Within a week of the TAVR procedure, he noticed significant improvements in his overall health:

1. He could ascend stairs without becoming breathless.
2. His energy levels noticeably increased, and he was free of chest discomfort.

The Importance of Early Detection

Mr Sharma's story is a wake-up call for anyone experiencing unexplained symptoms like fatigue or shortness of breath, especially if you're over sixty or have risk factors like smoking or a family history of heart disease. Early detection can save lives, and regular health check-ups – including echocardiograms when needed – are crucial.

Busting Common Misconceptions about TAVR

1. I'm too old for treatment: The reality is that TAVR is specifically designed for older adults and those at high risk. Age alone should not deter anyone from seeking treatment.
2. It is not as effective as surgery: Research indicates that TAVR is just as effective as traditional surgery for many patients, offering comparable long-term results.
3. Recovery will take months: Most patients who undergo TAVR return to their regular activities within a week of the procedure.

Who Can Benefit from TAVR?

1. Patients with severe aortic stenosis
2. Those who are too weak or high-risk for open-heart surgery
3. Older adults with other medical conditions that make surgery dangerous

How Long Does It Take?

The duration of a TAVR procedure typically ranges from 1 to 2 hours, but in some cases, such as this patient, the entire process can be completed in less than an hour. This quick procedure, combined with the reduced recovery time, makes TAVR an ideal option for high-risk patients.

The case highlights the life-saving potential of TAVR, offering hope to patients previously considered inoperable.

Why Is TAVR a Game Changer?

TAVR is a life-saving option for older patients or those who cannot undergo open-heart surgery due to their health conditions. It offers hope and a second chance at life for people who were previously considered too high-risk for surgery.

This seventy-six-year-old patient's journey is an incredible example of how modern medical advancements can completely change lives.

The Learning

Severe aortic stenosis should not be viewed as a death sentence, even in older individuals grappling with multiple health challenges. Thanks to innovations in medical technology like TAVR, people like Mr Sharma can look forward to a better quality of life with minimal risks and a short recovery period.

If you or someone you care about is experiencing symptoms like difficulty breathing or unusual fatigue, it is crucial not to disregard them. Engage in an open conversation with your doctor and discuss whether TAVR might be a viable option worth exploring.

Heart disease can happen without high cholesterol. Even if your cholesterol is normal, factors like inflammation, genetics and lifestyle can still cause heart disease.

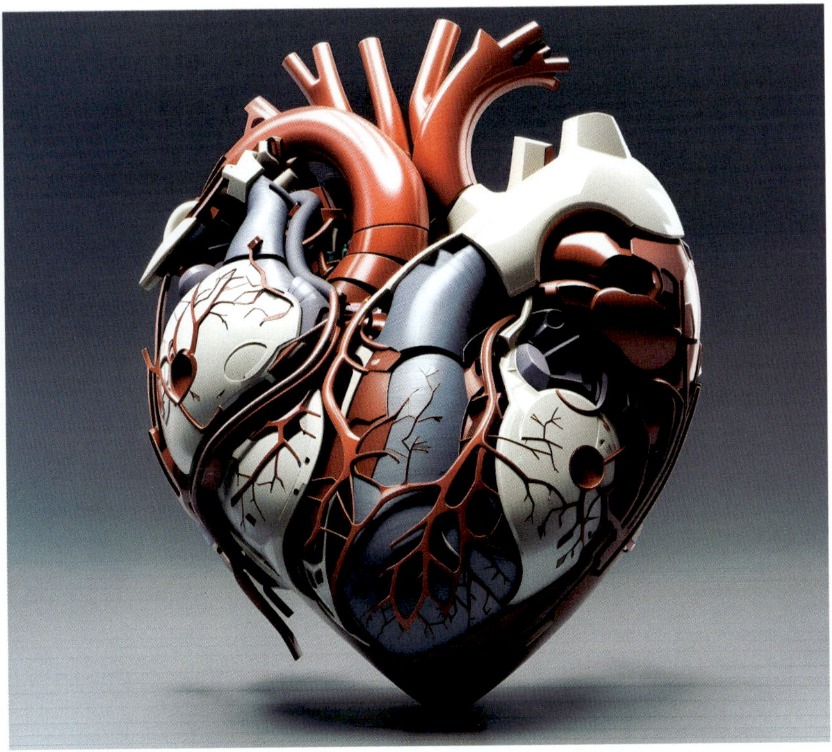

The heart: A symbol of life and health

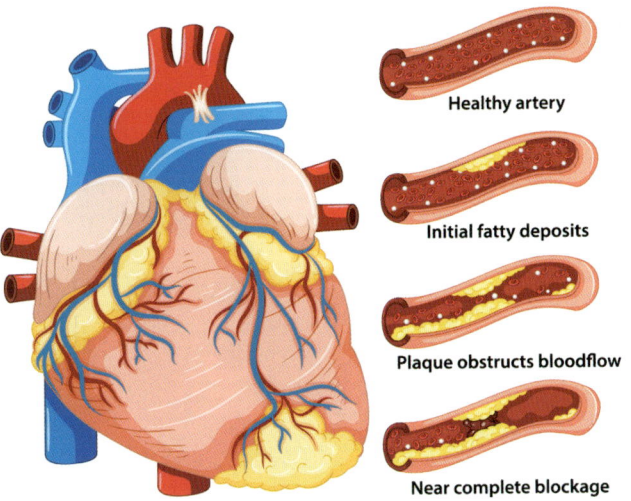

Beyond the first heart attack: Winning the fight against a second one

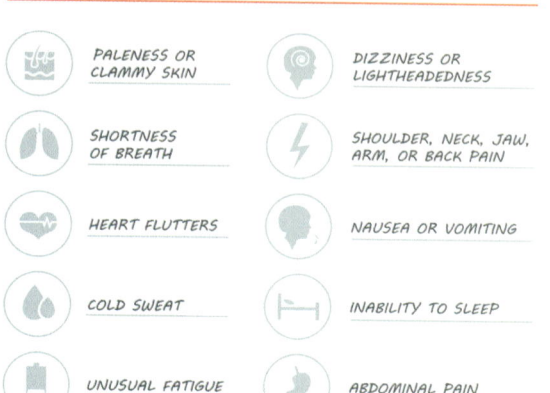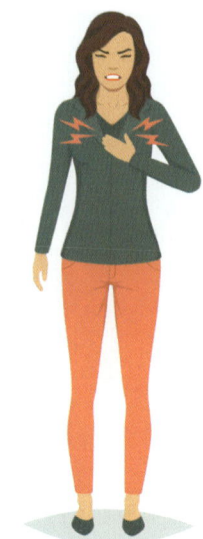

Not just chest pain: The subtle and often-missed heart attack signs in women

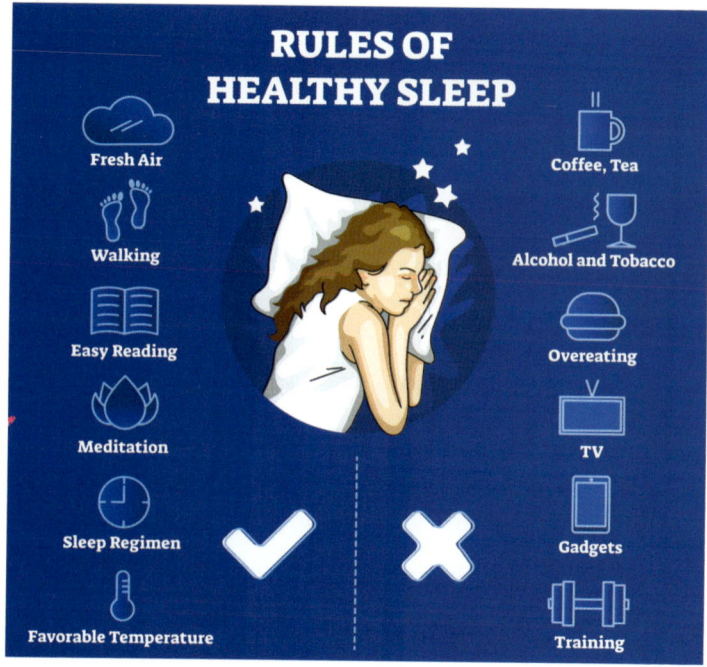

Master your sleep: The do's and don'ts for a perfect night's rest

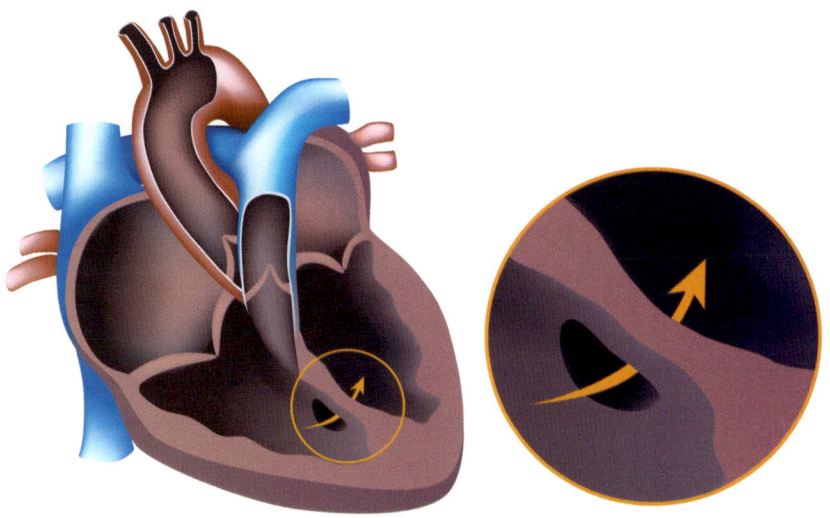

The hidden hole: A look inside a ventricular septal defect

Obstructive Sleep Apnoea Syndrome

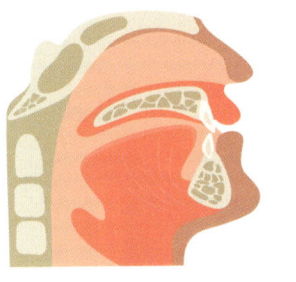

Normal
Breathing

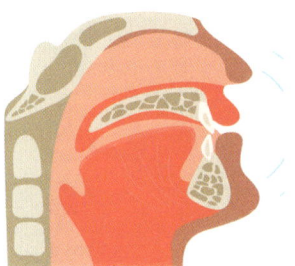

Snoring
(Partial Obstruction Of The Airway)

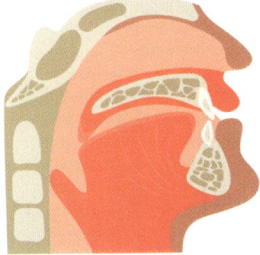

OSA
(Complete Obstruction Of The Airway)

More than just snoring: The serious health threat of sleep apnoea

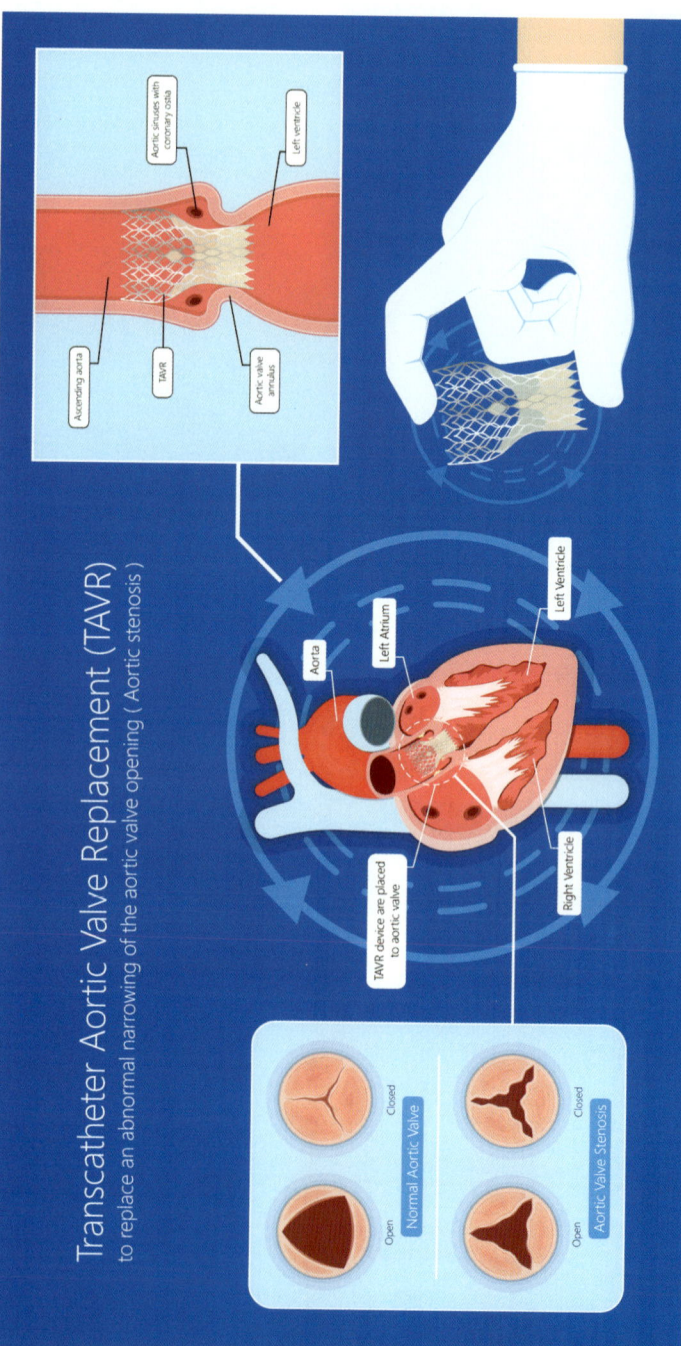

Fixing a failing valve without opening the chest: The breakthrough of Transcatheter Aortic Valve Replacement (TAVR)

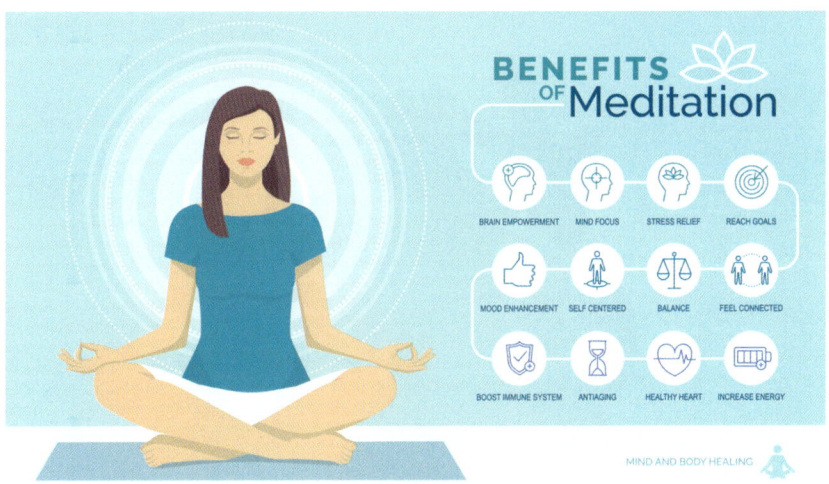

Why your brain needs meditation:
The surprising benefits for your mind, body and mood

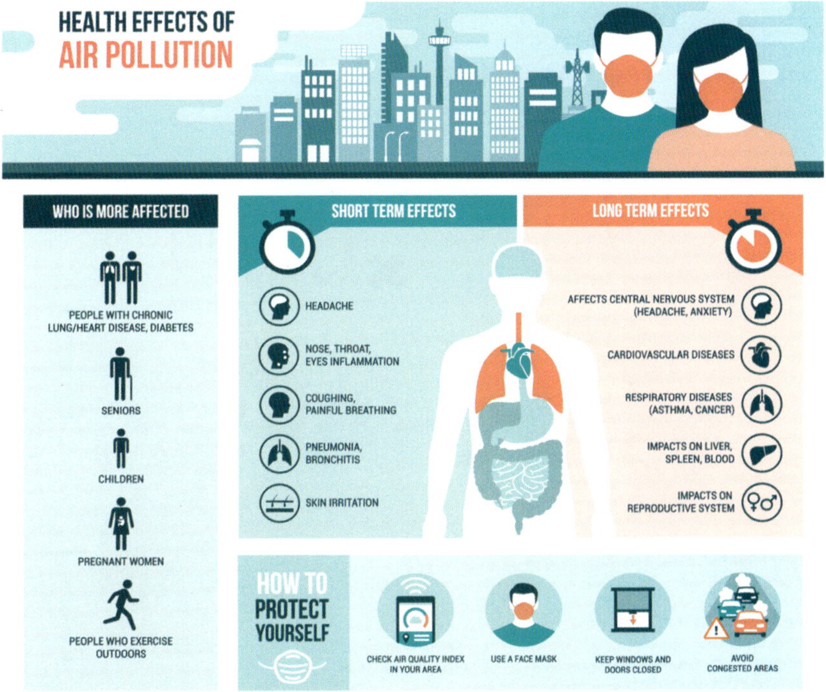

What are you really breathing? The short- and long-term toll of
air pollution on your health

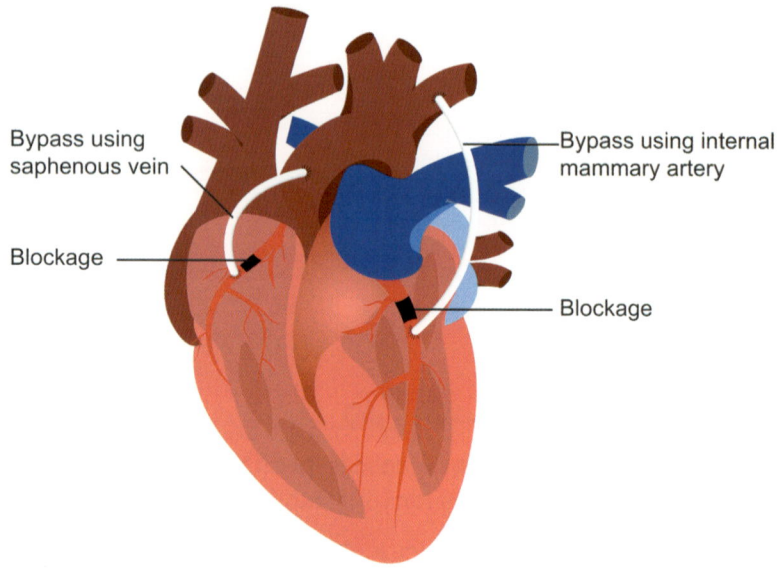

The heart's detour: Understanding single, double, triple and quadruple bypass surgery

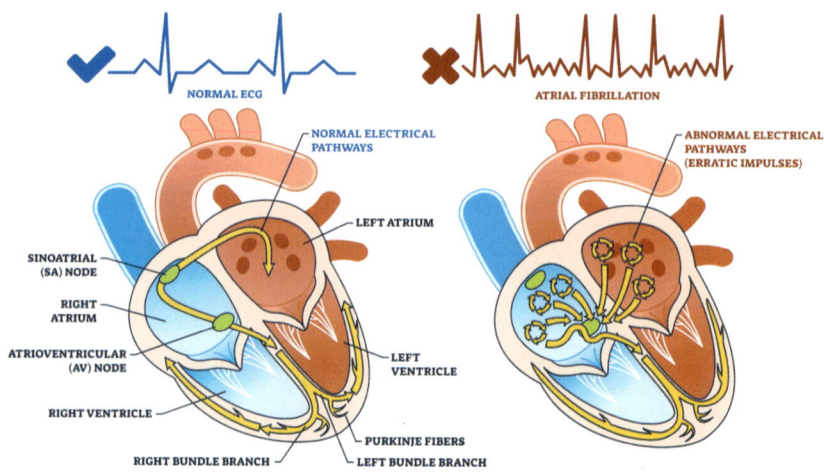

When your heart flutters instead of beating: Understanding atrial fibrillation

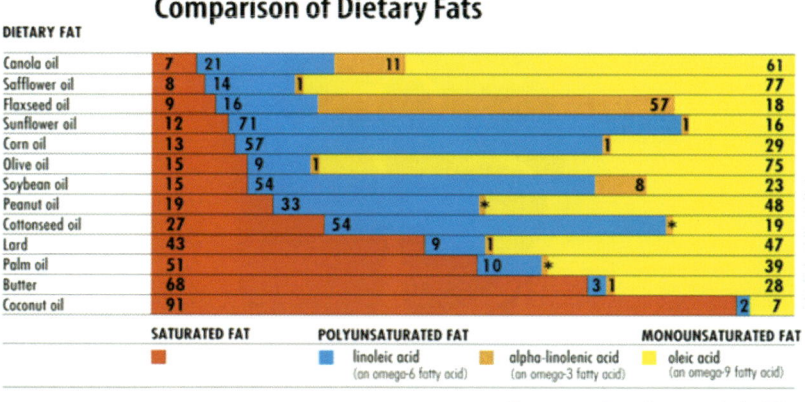

Good fats vs bad fats: A visual guide to making smarter choices

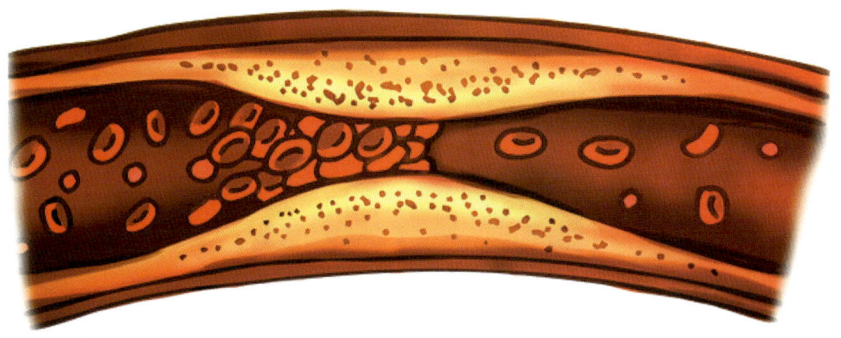

A ticking time bomb: Near-complete blockage obstructing blood flow

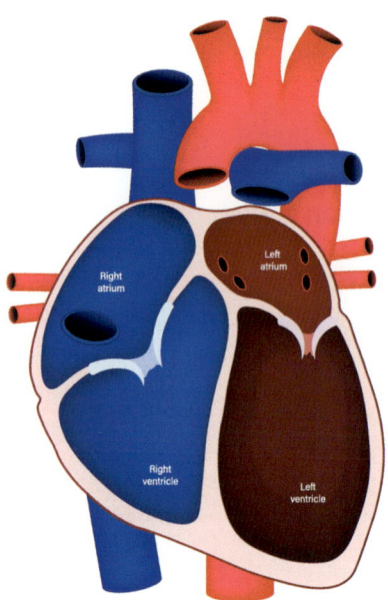

A normal heart

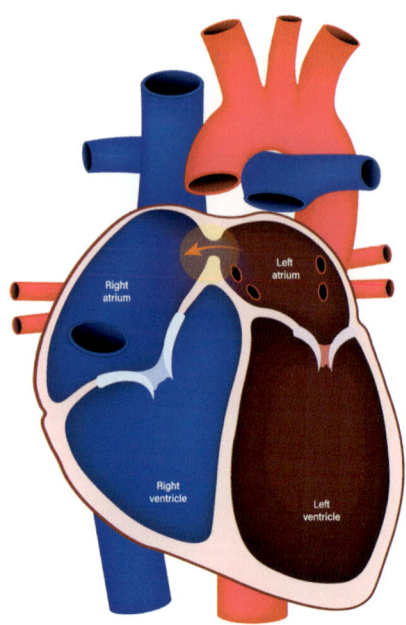

Atrial Septal Defect (ASD):
A hole between the heart's upper chambers

PART TWO

SCIENCE OF THE HEART: LIVING STRONGER, LIVING LONGER

24

Sleep and the Heart

SLEEP IS A VITAL component of overall health, particularly when it comes to maintaining cardiovascular well-being. Sleep is an essential process for the body, during which the body repairs and rejuvenates itself. During sleep, especially deep sleep stages like slow-wave sleep and rapid eye movement (REM) sleep, the body undergoes processes that help to regulate the immune system, support brain function and promote physical healing. One of the most vital functions of sleep is its ability to support heart health.

The relationship between sleep and heart health is multifaceted, with different stages of sleep, such as REM and NREM (non-rapid eye movement), playing distinct roles. Additionally, the advent of smartwatches and other wearable technology has enabled better sleep tracking and analysis, offering insights into how sleep quality affects heart health.

The Connection between Sleep and Heart Health

Sleep is not a passive state but rather a dynamic process during which the body undergoes various restorative functions. The heart, in particular, benefits from adequate sleep as it experiences a period of rest and recovery. However, disruptions in sleep, whether due to insufficient duration, poor quality or sleep disorders, can have detrimental effects on cardiovascular health.

Sleep Duration and Cardiovascular Risk

The duration of sleep has a direct impact on heart health. Studies have shown that adults who consistently sleep less than the recommended 7–8 hours per night are at a higher risk of developing cardiovascular diseases. Short sleep duration is associated with increased blood pressure, higher levels of stress hormones like cortisol and an elevated risk of conditions such as hypertension, CAD and heart failure. Conversely, excessive sleep (more than 9 hours) has also been linked to increased cardiovascular risk, though the reasons for this are less clear.

Sleep Quality and Heart Health

Sleep quality is just as important as sleep duration. Poor sleep quality, characterised by frequent awakenings or difficulty falling asleep, can lead to chronic inflammation, oxidative stress and dysregulation of the autonomic nervous system. These factors contribute to the development of atherosclerosis, arrhythmias and other cardiovascular conditions. For example, sleep disorders like obstructive sleep apnoea are strongly linked to hypertension, AFib and stroke.

REM and NREM Sleep: Their Role in Heart Health

Sleep is divided into two main stages: REM sleep and NREM sleep. Each of these stages plays a unique role in the body's recovery process and has specific implications for heart health.

NREM Sleep

NREM sleep, which accounts for about 75–80 per cent of total sleep time, is divided into three stages: N1, N2 and N3. During NREM sleep, the body's physiological processes slow down, allowing the heart and blood vessels to relax. The heart rate decreases, blood pressure drops and breathing becomes more regular. NREM sleep, particularly the deep N3 stage, is crucial for the body's physical restoration, including the repair of tissues and the strengthening of the immune system. This stage is also important for regulating blood sugar levels and reducing the risk of metabolic disorders that can negatively impact heart health.

REM Sleep

REM sleep is the stage of sleep where most dreaming occurs, and it accounts for about 20–25 per cent of total sleep time. During REM sleep, the brain is highly active, and the body experiences temporary muscle paralysis, with the exception of the eyes and respiratory muscles. Interestingly, during REM sleep, the heart rate and blood pressure can fluctuate more than during NREM sleep. While REM sleep is essential for cognitive functions like memory consolidation and emotional regulation, disruptions in REM sleep have been associated with an increased risk of cardiovascular events. For example, reduced REM sleep has been linked to a higher risk of developing hypertension and cardiovascular disease.

The Role of Smartwatches in Sleep Tracking and Sleep Analysis

With the rise of wearable technology, particularly smartwatches, individuals can now monitor their sleep patterns and gain insights into their sleep quality. These devices track various sleep metrics, including sleep duration, sleep stages (REM, NREM and light sleep) and the frequency of awakenings throughout the night.

Sleep Tracking Accuracy

While smartwatches are not as accurate as polysomnography (the gold standard for sleep studies), they offer a convenient and accessible way to monitor sleep. These devices use sensors to detect movement, heart rate and sometimes even blood oxygen levels, providing estimates of sleep stages and overall sleep quality. This data can help individuals identify patterns in their sleep and make informed decisions about lifestyle changes to improve sleep health.

Sleep Analysis and Heart Health

Smartwatches can also monitor heart rate variability during sleep, which is a key indicator of autonomic nervous system function and heart health. A higher heart rate variability is generally associated with better cardiovascular health and a well-functioning autonomic nervous system, while a lower variability can indicate stress, poor sleep quality and an increased risk of cardiovascular disease. By analysing sleep data over time, smartwatches can help identify trends that may indicate underlying health issues, such as sleep apnoea or insomnia, which are linked to cardiovascular risks.

Lifestyle Adjustments Based on Sleep Data

Armed with the information provided by smartwatches, individuals can make lifestyle adjustments to improve both sleep and heart health. For instance, they might establish a consistent sleep schedule, reduce caffeine intake or practise relaxation techniques before bed. Additionally, some smartwatches provide personalised sleep coaching, offering tips on how to improve sleep based on individual data.

Optimising Sleep for Heart Health

To maximise the benefits of sleep for heart health, consider the following tips.

1. Consistency is key: Aim to go to bed and wake up at the same time every day, even on weekends. This helps regulate the body's circadian rhythm and ensures high-quality sleep.
2. Create a sleep-friendly environment: Keep the bedroom cool, dark and quiet. Use blackout curtains and limit exposure to screens before bedtime as blue light can interfere with melatonin production.
3. Avoid stimulants: Refrain from consuming caffeine, alcohol or heavy meals late in the evening. These substances can disrupt sleep patterns and increase heart rate.

4. Address sleep apnoea: If you suspect you have sleep apnoea, consult a healthcare professional for evaluation and treatment options such as CPAP therapy.

The Learning

Sleep is an essential component of cardiovascular health, with both REM and NREM stages playing crucial roles in the body's restorative processes. Poor sleep, whether due to insufficient duration, poor quality or disrupted sleep stages, can significantly increase the risk of cardiovascular disease. The advent of smartwatches has made sleep tracking more accessible, allowing individuals to monitor their sleep patterns and make informed decisions about improving their sleep and heart health. By prioritising good sleep hygiene and utilising technology to track and analyse sleep, individuals can take proactive steps towards protecting their heart and overall well-being.

> Sleep deprivation increases heart attack risk. Less than 6 hours of sleep raises blood pressure, inflammation and heart disease risk.

25

Exercise and the Heart

OUR HEART AND EXERCISE are a team – one keeps us moving, and the other gets stronger with every step we take. In this chapter, we'll look at how staying active keeps our hearts happy and healthy. As numbers tell a story too, we'll also break down the math behind exercise and what it really means for our bodies. Let us get moving!

Debunking Myths about Exercise: How Much Is Too Much?

In an age where fitness culture dominates social media and wellness trends are ever-present, the question of how much exercise is too much has become increasingly relevant. While staying active is essential for maintaining good health, misconceptions about the right amount of exercise can lead to potential risks. We try to debunk common myths about exercise and clarify the fine line between beneficial physical activity and overtraining.

Myth 1: More Exercise Is Always Better

One of the most pervasive myths is that the more you exercise, the healthier you will be. While regular physical activity is crucial for cardiovascular health, weight management and mental well-being are also important. Over-exercising can lead to a range of health issues, including chronic fatigue, injuries, a weakened immune system and hormonal imbalances. These conditions can undermine the very health benefits that exercise is supposed to provide.

The key is balance. The American Heart Association recommends at least 150 minutes of moderate-intensity exercise or 75 minutes of vigorous-intensity exercise per week, combined with muscle-strengthening activities on two or more days a week.[1] Exceeding these recommendations occasionally can be beneficial for athletes or those training for specific events, but consistently pushing beyond these limits without adequate rest can lead to overtraining syndrome.

The 'milestone method' is a useful approach to balance exercise intensity and recovery. It emphasises milestones or specific goals within an exercise regimen, followed by periods of rest and active recovery. This method encourages setting achievable fitness goals, focusing on gradual progression and ensuring adequate rest to allow the body to repair and grow stronger. By following the milestone method, individuals can avoid the dangers of overtraining while still making steady progress towards their fitness goals.

Myth 2: Pain Is Just Part of the Process

The phrase 'no pain, no gain' has been a long-standing mantra in the fitness community. However, there is a significant difference between the discomfort of pushing your limits and the pain that signals injury. Ignoring the latter can result in long-term damage to muscles, tendons and joints. It is important to listen to your body and differentiate between normal muscle soreness and pain that may indicate overuse or strain.

Rest and recovery are crucial components of a well-rounded exercise regimen. Allowing your body to heal and adapt to the stress of exercise can prevent injuries and improve performance. Incorporating rest days and active recovery, such as light stretching or yoga, can help maintain the balance between staying active and avoiding burnout.

Myth 3: High-Intensity Training Is the Only Way to Get Results

High-intensity interval training has gained popularity for its efficiency and effectiveness in burning calories and building endurance. However, it is a myth that this is the only or best way to achieve fitness goals. While this type of training can be an excellent workout, especially for those with limited time, it is not suitable for everyone.

For some individuals, particularly beginners or those with certain health conditions, low- to moderate-intensity exercises like walking, cycling or swimming can be just as beneficial and pose fewer risks. Overdoing high-intensity workouts can increase the risk of cardiovascular events, especially if performed without proper warm-up or technique. A balanced fitness routine should include a mix of different intensities, depending on personal goals, fitness level and overall health.

Myth 4: You Need to Work Out Every Day

The idea that daily workouts are necessary for maintaining fitness is another common misconception. While consistency is important, rest days are equally vital. The body needs time to recover from the physical stress of exercise, rebuild muscle tissues and replenish energy stores. Over-exercising without allowing for proper recovery can lead to diminished performance, fatigue and even mental health challenges like anxiety and depression.

Aiming for three to five days of exercise per week, with rest or light activity on the other days, is generally sufficient for most people. This approach allows for physical improvements while minimising the risk of overuse injuries and burnout. Listening to your body and adjusting your workout schedule based on how you feel can also help in maintaining long-term fitness without overdoing it.

Myth 5: Exercise Can Offset Poor Lifestyle Choices

Many people believe that intense exercise can compensate for unhealthy habits like poor diet, inadequate sleep or excessive stress. While exercise is an important component of a healthy lifestyle, it cannot completely counteract the negative effects of these habits. Optimal health requires a holistic approach that includes balanced nutrition, sufficient rest, stress management and regular physical activity.

Myth 6: Switching Off Air Conditioning Enhances Workout Benefits

Some fitness enthusiasts believe that working out without air conditioning will increase sweat production, leading to greater calorie burn and detoxification. However, this is a myth that can pose significant health risks. While sweating is a natural cooling mechanism, it does not necessarily indicate increased fat burning. Excessive sweating in a hot environment can lead to dehydration, heat exhaustion or even heatstroke.

Turning off the AC during a workout may make you feel like you're working harder, but it doesn't translate to more significant fitness gains. In hot and humid conditions, your body's ability to cool itself is compromised, which can result in an elevated heart rate and decreased performance. To maximise workout efficiency and safety, maintain a comfortable temperature, stay hydrated and focus on the quality of your exercise routine rather than sweating excessively.

Myth 7: Supplements, Steroids and Hormones Are a Shortcut to Fitness

The fitness industry is flooded with products promising quick results, including supplements, steroids and hormones. While some supplements, such as protein powders, vitamins and minerals, can support a balanced diet and help meet nutritional needs, others can be harmful if misused.

Good Supplements

Protein supplements can aid in muscle recovery, creatine can enhance strength and performance, and branched-chain amino acids can reduce muscle soreness. However, these should be used as part of a well-rounded diet and under the guidance of a healthcare professional.

Risks of Steroids and Hormones

The misuse of anabolic steroids and hormones like testosterone can lead to serious health issues, including heart disease, liver damage, hormonal imbalances and psychological effects such as aggression and depression. While these substances can lead to rapid muscle growth and performance enhancement, the long-term risks far outweigh the short-term benefits. Additionally, the use of such substances without medical supervision is illegal and can lead to severe legal consequences.

The best approach to fitness is natural, emphasising a balanced diet, regular exercise and adequate rest. Supplements can be beneficial when used correctly, but they are not a substitute for hard work, dedication and a healthy lifestyle.

Target Heart Rate: Understanding the Phases

Monitoring your heart rate during exercise is an effective way to ensure you're working out at the right intensity. The target heart rate is a range that reflects the optimal intensity for cardiovascular exercise. It is typically calculated as a percentage of your maximum heart rate, which can be estimated by subtracting your age from 220.

The target heart rate can be broken down into different phases:

Warm-Up Phase (50–60 Per Cent of Maximum Heart Rate)

This phase prepares your body for exercise, gradually increasing your heart rate and loosening your muscles. Warm-up is essential for reducing the risk of injury and ensuring that your body is ready for more intense activity.

Fat-Burning Phase (60–70 Per Cent of Maximum Heart Rate)

In this phase, your body efficiently burns fat for energy. It is ideal for those aiming to lose weight and improve endurance. The exercise intensity is moderate, allowing you to sustain activity for longer periods.

Aerobic Phase (70–80 Per Cent of Maximum Heart Rate)

This phase focuses on improving cardiovascular fitness and endurance. It is a moderate to high-intensity phase where the body uses both fat and carbohydrates for energy. Regularly exercising in this zone can improve heart health and increase lung capacity.

Anaerobic Phase (80–90 Per Cent of Maximum Heart Rate)

This phase is for building strength, speed and power. It involves short bursts of high-intensity exercise, where the body primarily uses carbohydrates for energy. While effective for building muscle and improving athletic performance, this phase should be approached cautiously to avoid overtraining.

Maximum Effort Phase (90–100 Per Cent of Maximum Heart Rate)

This phase represents the highest intensity level, used for short sprints or high-intensity interval training. It is not sustainable for long periods and should only be attempted by those with a high fitness level and under proper supervision.

The Learning

Exercise is a vital component of a healthy lifestyle but must be approached with knowledge and balance. The milestone method offers a structured way to progress in fitness without risking overtraining. Maintaining a comfortable environment, including using air conditioning, can prevent heat-related illnesses during workouts. While supplements can support your fitness goals, steroids and hormones carry significant risks that should not be overlooked. Finally, understanding and monitoring your target heart rate phases ensures that you're exercising effectively and safely.

Exercise is undoubtedly a key pillar of good health, but more isn't always better. Understanding the balance between physical activity, rest and recovery is essential for achieving and maintaining fitness goals. Dispelling these myths about exercise can help individuals adopt a more informed and balanced approach to their fitness journey, reducing the risk of overtraining and promoting long-term well-being.

> Exercise can cause heart attacks – if you do it wrong. Intense workouts in untrained individuals or without proper warm-up can trigger heart attacks.

26

Pollution and the Heart

ENVIRONMENTAL POLLUTION IS A growing global health concern with significant implications for cardiovascular health. In India, the rapid pace of urbanisation and industrialisation has led to alarming levels of air pollution in many metropolitan areas. The link between air pollution and heart health has been increasingly recognised, with pollutants such as particulate matter (PM), nitrogen dioxide (NO_2), sulphur dioxide (SO_2), carbon monoxide (CO) and ozone (O_3) playing a pivotal role in the development and progression of cardiovascular diseases. This chapter explores how these pollutants impact heart health, the pollution levels in various metro cities in India and the precise measures that can be taken to prevent the adverse effects of pollution on the heart.

How Environmental Pollution Affects Heart Health

Particulate Matter (PM2.5 and PM10)

Particulate matter, particularly PM2.5 and PM10, is one of the most significant contributors to air pollution and a major threat to heart health. PM2.5 particles, which are smaller than 2.5 micrometres in diameter, can penetrate deep into the lungs, enter the bloodstream and cause systemic inflammation. This inflammation leads to endothelial dysfunction, a condition where the inner lining of blood vessels doesn't function properly, increasing the risk of atherosclerosis. Atherosclerosis can lead to CAD, heart attacks and strokes. In India, high levels of PM2.5

are associated with an increased incidence of hypertension, heart failure and arrhythmias.

NO_2

NO_2, primarily produced from vehicle emissions and industrial activities, is another critical pollutant affecting heart health. When inhaled, NO_2 causes oxidative stress, which damages the endothelial cells lining the arteries. This damage promotes the formation of atherosclerotic plaques (atherosclerosis) and increases blood pressure, both of which are significant risk factors for heart attacks and strokes. Chronic exposure to high levels of NO_2 can lead to the progression of heart failure and increase the likelihood of sudden cardiac events.

SO_2

SO_2 is produced from the burning of fossil fuels, such as coal and oil, and is prevalent in industrial areas. When inhaled, SO_2 causes bronchoconstriction, which increases the workload on the heart by reducing oxygen supply and causing systemic inflammation. This can exacerbate conditions such as CAD, leading to heart attacks. Short-term spikes in SO_2 levels have been linked to increased hospital admissions for cardiovascular events, particularly in individuals with pre-existing heart conditions.

CO

CO, a byproduct of incomplete combustion, is a colourless, odourless gas that binds with haemoglobin in the blood much more readily than oxygen. This binding reduces the oxygen-carrying capacity of the blood, leading to hypoxia (oxygen deficiency). The heart, being highly sensitive to oxygen levels, can suffer significant damage due to CO exposure. In patients with existing heart disease, even low levels of CO exposure can trigger angina and arrhythmias and increase the risk of myocardial infarction (heart attack).

O_3

O_3 is a secondary pollutant formed by the reaction of sunlight with pollutants such as NO_2 and volatile organic compounds. It is a potent respiratory and cardiovascular irritant. Acute exposure to high O_3 levels can cause oxidative stress and inflammation in the cardiovascular system, leading to an increased risk of heart attacks, strokes and worsening heart failure. Chronic exposure has been associated with the development of atherosclerosis and other cardiovascular conditions.

Pollution Levels in Various Metro Cities in India

India's metro cities are some of the most polluted in the world, with air quality frequently falling below safe standards. Here's a look at pollution levels in key Indian metros:

1. Delhi: Delhi consistently ranks as one of the most polluted cities globally with PM2.5 levels often exceeding 150 μg/m^3, especially during winter months when crop burning and temperature inversions worsen air quality. The city also faces high levels of NO_2 and CO, primarily due to heavy traffic and industrial activities.[1]
2. Mumbai: Mumbai, while slightly better off than Delhi, still faces serious pollution challenges, particularly with PM2.5 levels ranging from 40 to 70 μg/m^3. The city's pollution is driven by traffic emissions, construction activities and industrial discharges.[2]
3. Kolkata: Kolkata experiences PM2.5 levels that frequently exceed 60 μg/m^3, along with high concentrations of NO_2 and SO_2 due to vehicular emissions and industrial pollution.[3]
4. Chennai: Chennai faces moderate to high levels of PM2.5, often ranging between 30 and 60 μg/m^3. The city's air pollution is largely driven by vehicular emissions and industrial activities, with significant contributions from NO_2 and SO_2.[4]

5. Bengaluru: Bengaluru, while known for its relatively better air quality, still faces rising levels of PM2.5, particularly during the dry months. PM2.5 levels in the city range from 30 to 50 µg/m^3.[5]

These pollution levels contribute to a significant burden of cardiovascular disease, with higher rates of hypertension, heart attacks and strokes observed in the population.

Preventive Measures to Protect Heart Health

Reducing Personal Exposure

Individuals should take steps to minimise exposure to air pollution, particularly on days when air quality is poor. This includes staying indoors during peak pollution times, using air purifiers at home and wearing masks when outdoor activities are necessary. Regular monitoring of air quality through apps can help individuals plan their activities to reduce exposure.

Advocating for Cleaner Air Policies

Public health advocacy is crucial in addressing the root causes of air pollution. This includes supporting stricter emission standards for vehicles, promoting the use of clean energy and pushing for the implementation of pollution control measures in industrial sectors. Cardiologists and healthcare professionals can play a key role in these advocacy efforts by highlighting the link between air pollution and cardiovascular disease.

Encouraging Lifestyle Modifications

Adopting a healthy lifestyle can mitigate some of the harmful effects of pollution on the heart. This includes maintaining a diet rich in antioxidants, which can help combat oxidative stress caused by pollution. Regular physical activity is also important, although it should be done indoors when outdoor air quality is poor. Giving up smoking is particularly crucial as smoking compounds the cardiovascular risks associated with air pollution.

Regular Health Monitoring

For individuals living in high-pollution areas, regular cardiovascular check-ups are essential. Monitoring blood pressure, cholesterol levels and other cardiovascular markers can help detect early signs of pollution-related heart issues. Healthcare providers should consider pollution exposure when assessing cardiovascular risk and tailor preventive strategies accordingly.

The Learning

Environmental pollution is a significant threat to heart health, particularly in India's metro cities where pollution levels are alarmingly high. Pollutants such as PM2.5, NO_2, SO_2, CO and O_3 contribute to the development and exacerbation of cardiovascular diseases, leading to increased morbidity and mortality. However, by reducing personal exposure, advocating for cleaner air policies, encouraging lifestyle modifications and ensuring regular health monitoring, the adverse effects of pollution on heart health can be mitigated.

> Air pollution is a major cause of heart disease. Fine particles (PM2.5) from pollution enter the bloodstream, causing inflammation and blockages.

27

Food and Heart Health

WHEN IT COMES TO keeping your heart healthy, what you eat plays a huge role – and the types of oils you use in your kitchen are more important than you might think. Oils are a part of our daily meals, whether it is a drizzle on salad or a base for frying. However, not all oils are created equal. Some support your heart, helping it stay strong and disease-free, while others do the exact opposite.

Let us break down the kinds of fats in oils, which ones are good or bad for your heart, the best oils to use and how you can make smart choices.

Types of Fats in Oils

Oils can contain different types of fats, and each has a unique effect on heart health.

Unsaturated Fats

Unsaturated fats are beneficial for heart health. They are the healthy fats your body actually needs. They are found in many plant-based oils and some fish. There are two types of healthy unsaturated fats:

1. Monounsaturated fats (MUFA): Found in olive oil, canola oil, peanut oil and avocados, these fats help reduce bad cholesterol (LDL) and maintain good cholesterol (HDL), improving overall heart health. They're a great everyday choice for cooking and salad dressings.

2. Polyunsaturated fats (PUFA): These fats are found in sunflower oil, corn oil and fish oils. Omega-3 fatty acids, a type of PUFA found in fish oil and flaxseeds, are especially beneficial for reducing inflammation and the risk of arrhythmias, lowering triglycerides and preventing heart disease.

Saturated Fats

Saturated fats are less heart-healthy and must be used with caution. They are found in coconut oil, palm oil, butter and animal fats. A high intake of saturated fats can raise LDL cholesterol, increasing the risk of atherosclerosis, heart attack and stroke. However, recent studies suggest that some saturated fats, such as those in coconut oil, may have a neutral effect, though moderation is still key.[1]

Trans Fats

Trans fats are the troublemakers. These fats are the worst for your heart. They are found in partially hydrogenated oils, which are used in processed and fried foods. Trans fats significantly increase LDL cholesterol and reduce HDL cholesterol, greatly increasing the risk of heart disease and stroke. These should be avoided as much as possible.

Key Oils for Heart Health: The Best Choices for Everyday Use

Let us look at some of the healthiest oils you can add to your diet – and why they're so good for your heart.

Olive Oil (Extra-Virgin)

Olive oil is the staple of the Mediterranean diet, which is one of the healthiest diets in the world. Extra-virgin olive oil is full of healthy fats and antioxidants that help protect your heart. It can lower bad cholesterol and improve how your blood vessels work – all of which help prevent heart disease. It also has anti-inflammatory properties that help protect against atherosclerosis.

Canola Oil

This oil has a good mix of healthy fats, including omega-3s and omega-6s. It is low in bad fats and helps keep cholesterol levels in a healthy range. It is also great for cooking at different temperatures, making it very versatile.

Flaxseed Oil

Flaxseed oil is rich in omega-3 fatty acids, which can help lower blood pressure, reduce swelling and improve cholesterol levels. It is best used in dressings or added to food after cooking because it isn't good for high heat.

Fish Oil

Fish oil supplements or eating fatty fish like salmon or mackerel is one of the best ways to get omega-3 fatty acids, particularly eicosapentaenoic acid (EPA) and docosahexaenoic acid (DHA). These healthy fats can help reduce fat in the blood (triglycerides), lower blood pressure and cut your risk of heart attacks and strokes.

Coconut Oil

Despite being high in saturated fat, coconut oil has gained popularity. Its effects on heart health are still debated, though it appears to raise both HDL and LDL cholesterol. It is best used in moderation and as part of a balanced diet.

Guidelines for Eating Oils the Heart-Healthy Way

Even Good Oils Should Be Used in Moderation

Just because an oil is healthy doesn't mean you can pour it on everything. Oils are still high in calories. So, using too much can lead to weight gain, which is a risk factor for heart disease.

Food and Heart Health

Balance of Omega-3 and Omega-6

While both are essential, an imbalance with too much omega-6 (found in oils like corn and sunflower) can promote inflammation. Omega-3-rich oils (fish oil, flaxseed) should be prioritised to counterbalance this effect.

Choose the Right Oil for Cooking

Different oils react differently to heat. When cooking at high temperatures, like frying, use oils with a high smoke point, such as canola oil or avocado oil, to avoid harmful compounds that can form when oils are overheated.

Say Goodbye to Trans Fats

Avoid packaged snacks and fried fast foods that are high in trans fats. Look at labels for the words *partially hydrogenated oil* and steer clear. Instead, choose natural oils like olive, canola or flaxseed.

Oils and Common Heart Issues: How the Right Oils Can Help

1. High blood pressure (hypertension): Oils like fish oil and flaxseed oil that are high in omega-3s can help bring down blood pressure, taking the pressure off your heart.
2. Clogged arteries (atherosclerosis): Oils like olive oil, which have antioxidants and anti-inflammatory benefits, can help prevent plaque build-up in your arteries and reduce the risk of atherosclerosis.
3. Unhealthy blood fat levels (dyslipidaemia): Unsaturated fats (from olive oil, fish oil and the like) can help lower bad fats (like LDL and triglycerides) and raise good fats (HDL) in your blood. This lowers the risk of heart disease.

A Heart-Healthy Diet: It Is More than Just Oil

A heart-healthy diet includes a balance of healthy oils, whole grains, lean proteins (fish, poultry), fruits and vegetables. The

Mediterranean diet is one of the best examples, with an emphasis on olive oil, fish, nuts and plant-based foods. Intake of processed foods, refined carbohydrates and foods high in saturated and trans fats must be limited as these can contribute to obesity, diabetes and heart disease.

The Learning

Choosing the right oils can make a big difference in your heart's health. Oils that are rich in unsaturated fats, such as olive oil, canola oil, flaxseed oil and fish oil, help protect your heart and keep your blood vessels working well. At the same time, you should avoid harmful trans fats and limit saturated fats.

Remember, balance is everything. Don't go overboard – even healthy oils should be used in moderation. Aim for a mix of good fats, eat a variety of wholesome foods and keep your lifestyle active. Your heart will thank you for it.

> Omega-3 sources for vegetarians are walnuts, linseeds (flaxseeds), chia seeds, oils and spreads.

28

Hearty Recipes

FOOD IS MORE THAN just sustenance – it is the heart's closest ally. Every bite we take has the power to nourish, protect and strengthen the very organ that keeps us going. In this chapter, we bring you ten carefully curated, heart-healthy recipes that not only prioritise nutrition but also celebrate flavour. Whether you're looking for a comforting meal, a refreshing salad or a satisfying snack, these recipes strike the perfect balance between taste and wellness. Packed with wholesome ingredients, essential nutrients and vibrant flavours, each dish is designed to support heart health without compromising on indulgence.

These recipes have been thoughtfully curated by Sobana Laxmi Jagraj, a holistic nutritionist, who makes healthy eating an effortless part of everyday life. With a deep passion for experimenting with wholesome ingredients and mindful cooking techniques, she transforms nutritious meals into something truly enjoyable. Her approach isn't about rigid diets but about creating lasting, sustainable habits that support overall well-being. Through these recipes, she invites you to embrace a way of eating that is both heart-friendly and deeply satisfying.

Oats and Vegetable Soup

Serving size: 4
Preparation time: 10 minutes
Cooking time: 10 minutes

Ingredients
Mixed vegetables: 1 cup, bite-size cut (beans, celery, cabbage, carrots, leeks, spinach)
Rolled oats: 2 tbsp
Garlic: 1 tbsp, finely chopped
Onions: ¼ cup, finely chopped
Coriander leaves: 2 tbsp, chopped
Water: 3 cups
Salt and pepper to taste

Procedure
Chop the vegetables into bite-sized pieces. Sauté the garlic, onions and the chopped mixed vegetables in 1 teaspoon of oil on a medium flame for 3-5 minutes until softened. Pour in 3 cups of water to cover the vegetables and cook on a medium flame for 2 minutes. After 2 minutes, add oats and the chopped coriander leaves. Bring the mixture to a boil, then reduce the heat and let it simmer for 20-30 minutes to blend the flavours. Add salt and pepper for extra flavour. Serve oats and vegetable soup hot, and enjoy your healthy and tasty soup.

Roasted Pumpkin Soup

Serving size: 2
Preparation time: 10 minutes
Cooking time: 30 minutes

Ingredients
Pumpkin/butternut squash: 200 g
Garlic: 2 cloves
Oil: Spray as needed
Onion: ½, diced
Carrot: 1 large, chopped
Celery stalk: 1, chopped
Chilli powder: ¾ tsp

Cumin powder: ¼ tsp
Olive oil: 1 tsp
Salt and pepper to taste
Home-made low-sodium vegetable broth/water: 1¼ cups

Procedure
Preheat your oven to 400°F (200°C). Place the pumpkin and garlic cloves on a baking sheet. Spray with oil. Roast for 25–30 minutes until the pumpkin is tender. In a pot, heat olive oil over medium heat. Add the onion, carrot and celery. Sauté for 5–7 minutes until softened. Add chilli powder, cumin powder, roasted pumpkin and the roasted garlic (peeled). Stir well. Pour in the veggie broth/water, bringing it to a boil. Reduce the heat and simmer for 15 minutes. Blend the soup until smooth using an immersion blender. Season with salt and pepper to taste. Serve the soup hot, topped with a tablespoon of Greek yoghurt for a creamy finish.

Note: For a crunchy feel, you can chop and sprinkle walnuts or almonds on top.

Broccoli Almond Soup

Serving size: 4
Preparation time: 10 minutes
Cooking time: 25 minutes
Ingredients
Olive oil: 1 tsp
Onion: 1 medium, finely chopped
Garlic cloves: 3, minced
Ginger: 2-inch piece, minced
Coriander stems: 20, chopped
Almonds: 20, blanched and peeled
Water: 1 litre
Salt to taste
Broccoli: 250 g, chopped

Black pepper: ½ tsp
Vegetable stock: 1½ cups (adjust as needed)
Toasted almonds: For garnish, cut into thin slivers

Method
Heat olive oil in a large pan over medium heat. Add chopped onion, garlic and ginger. Sauté until the onion turns translucent. Stir in the coriander stems and almonds. Sauté for 2 minutes until fragrant. Pour in 1 litre of water and add salt to taste. Bring to a boil, then add chopped broccoli. Cover and cook for 10 minutes until the broccoli becomes tender. Strain the stock and set it aside. Allow them to cool. Blend the cooked vegetables until smooth. Return the purée to the pan. Add black pepper and 1½ cups of vegetable stock (or adjust as per desired consistency). Bring the soup to a gentle boil twice. Taste test for salt, and adjust seasoning if necessary. Serve hot, garnished with a sprinkle of black pepper and toasted almonds for crunch. Enjoy this wholesome and heart-healthy soup!

Black *Chana* (Chickpeas) and Sweet Potato Salad

Serving size: 3
Preparation time: 15 minutes
Ingredients
Black chana: 200 g, pressure cooked to soft
Sweet potatoes: 200 g, peeled and steamed
Avocados: 2, diced
Corn kernels: ¼ cup, boiled
Red bell pepper: 1, diced
Onion: ¼ cup, chopped
Fresh cilantro: ¼ cup, chopped
Lime juice to taste
Chilli powder: ½ tsp
Salt and pepper to taste
Pomegranate seeds for sprinkling on top

Procedure
Add the pressure-cooked black chana, steamed sweet potato, boiled corn, red bell pepper, onion and cilantro to a large salad bowl. Squeeze the limes over the top, and add the chilli powder. Season with salt and black pepper to taste, and then toss the salad until it is fully coated. Taste the salad and adjust the seasonings, lime juice, salt and pepper if needed. Cover the salad and let it chill in the refrigerator for 30 minutes to 1 hour. Right before serving, top each individual bowl with diced avocado and sprinkle with pomegranate seeds. Serve with extra lime wedges on the side, if desired.

Green Papaya Salad

Servings: 4
Preparation time: 20 minutes

Ingredients
Garlic clove: 2 small, minced
Thai chillies: 2 to 3, finely chopped
Unsalted peanuts: 2 tbsp, roasted and divided
Cherry tomatoes: 4, halved
Long beans: 2 (about 30 g), trimmed and cut into 2-inch pieces
Apple cider vinegar: 1 tbsp
Green papaya: 150 g, shredded
Salt to taste

Procedure
In a mixing bowl, combine the minced garlic and chopped Thai chillies. Lightly crush them with the back of a spoon to release their flavours. Add 1 tablespoon of the roasted peanuts and the halved cherry tomatoes. Gently press them with the spoon to release the tomato juices. Toss in the long beans, and lightly bruise them with the spoon until they are slightly tender. Pour in the apple cider vinegar, and sprinkle with salt to taste. Mix well until the ingredients

are coated. Add the shredded green papaya and toss thoroughly to combine, ensuring the dressing coats the papaya evenly. Sprinkle the remaining tablespoon of peanuts over the salad. Transfer to a serving plate, and enjoy it fresh.

Avocado Chia Overnight Oats Recipe

Servings: 2
Preparation time: 10 minutes
Refrigeration time: 4 hours or overnight

Ingredients
Chia seeds: 2 tbsp
Rolled oats: 2 tbsp
Pumpkin seeds: 1 tbsp (optional)
Almond milk or low-fat dairy milk: ¾ cup
Fruit of choice (for example, ½ cup sliced banana, strawberries, blueberries or diced mango)
Toppings of choice (for example, 2 tbsp peanut butter, Greek yoghurt or chopped nuts such as almonds, walnuts or hazelnuts)
Ripe avocado: ⅓ cup, mashed
Cinnamon powder: ½ tsp
Brown sugar to taste

Procedure
In a bowl or jar, combine chia seeds, rolled oats and pumpkin seeds (if using). In a separate bowl, mash the avocado until smooth. Add almond milk or low-fat dairy, cinnamon powder and brown sugar. Mix until creamy and well blended. Pour the avocado and milk mixture into the chia and oat mixture. Ensure that all ingredients are fully immersed in the liquid to allow even absorption and stir thoroughly to coat everything evenly. Cover and refrigerate for at least 4 hours or overnight until thickened. Before serving, give the mixture a good stir. Add your choice of fruit, and top with your favourite toppings like peanut butter, Greek yoghurt

or chopped nuts. Serve chilled for a creamy, nutrient-packed breakfast or snack!

Dalia Khichdi

Serving size: 2
Preparation time: 10 minutes
Cooking time: 15 minutes

Ingredients
Daliya/broken wheat: ½ cup
Moong dal: ¼ cup
Cold-pressed mustard oil: 1 tsp
Mustard seeds: 1 tsp
Cumin seeds: 1 tsp
Asafoetida: 1 pinch
Dried red chilli: 1
Curry leaves: A few
Carrot: 1, chopped
Beans: ½ cup, chopped
Peas: 2 tbsp
Tomato: 1, chopped
Ginger paste: ½ tsp
Turmeric powder: ¼ tsp
Kashmiri red chilli powder: ¾ tsp
Garam masala: ½ tsp
Salt to taste
Water: 3 cups
Coriander leaves: 2 tbsp, finely chopped

Procedure
In a large bowl, take ½ cup broken wheat and ¼ cup moong dal. Soak them in enough water for 10 minutes. After soaking, drain the water. In a pressure cooker, heat 1 tsp of mustard oil over medium heat. Once the oil is hot, add 1 tsp mustard seeds and

1 tsp cumin seeds. Let them splutter. Add a pinch of asafoetida, 1 dried red chilli and a few curry leaves. Sauté for a few seconds. Add the drained broken wheat and moong dal to the tempering. Sauté for 2 minutes until the mixture becomes aromatic. Lower the heat, and add ¼ tsp turmeric powder, ¾ tsp Kashmiri red chilli powder, ½ tsp garam masala and ¾ tsp salt. Stir well, and sauté for 1 minute to combine the spices. Add ginger paste, and sauté well for a minute. Add chopped tomatoes, and sauté them until they become mushy. Next add the vegetables: chopped carrot, chopped beans and peas. Pour in 3 cups of water, and stir everything together. Close the lid of the pressure cooker, and cook for three whistles or until the broken wheat and moong dal are fully cooked and softened. Once the pressure settles, open the cooker, and add 2 tbsp finely chopped coriander. Stir well, and adjust the consistency by adding more water if needed. Serve the warm khichdi with a vegetable raita for a complete and hearty meal.

Shredded Chicken and Avocado Spaghetti

Serving size: 4
Preparation time: 15 minutes
Cooking time: 15 minutes

Ingredients
Parsley leaves: 1 cup, firmly packed
Onions: 1, thinly sliced
Lemon rind: 2 tsp
Lemon juice: ¼ cup
Avocado: 1 large, halved
Cooked shredded chicken: 450 g
Wholemeal spaghetti: 200 g
Green olives: ¼ cup, sliced
Baby rocket leaves: 60 g
Toasted almonds: 1 tbsp, chopped

Olive oil: 1 tsp
Almonds: 5, toasted and chopped
Salt and pepper to taste

Procedure
Blend the parsley, onions, lemon rind and lemon juice in a food processor until finely chopped. Add half of the avocado, and pulse to form a smooth paste. In a frying pan, add olive oil, and cook the shredded chicken over medium heat for about 5–7 minutes until it is heated through and slightly crispy. Remove from the pan and set aside. Meanwhile, cook the wholemeal spaghetti in a large saucepan of boiling water following the packet directions. Reserve ½ cup of pasta water, and then drain the spaghetti.

In a large bowl, add the cooked spaghetti and reserved pasta water. Next, add the cooked, shredded chicken, avocado paste, sliced olives and rocket leaves. Season with freshly ground pepper and salt to taste, and toss gently to combine. Serve the spaghetti into serving bowls. Top with thinly sliced avocado, and sprinkle with chopped toasted almonds.

Horse Gram Chutney

Serves: 4
Preparation time: 10 minutes
Cooking time: 10 minutes

Ingredients
Horse gram: 1 tbsp
Red chillies: 3
Tamarind: 10 g
Oil: 1 tsp
Small onions: 12
Tomato: 1, chopped
Garlic: 2–3 flakes
Curry leaves: 6

Mustard seeds: ¼ tsp
Urad dal (black gram split): ¼ tsp
Salt to taste

Procedure
In a pan, heat ½ tsp of oil. Add horse gram, red chillies and tamarind. Sauté on low flame until the horse gram pops. Remove from the pan, and set aside. In the same pan, add peeled small onions and garlic. Cook until the small onions turn golden brown. Add chopped tomatoes, and sauté until they become mushy. Add curry leaves, and switch off the flame. Stir in salt to taste. Allow the mixture to cool completely. Once cooled, grind the mixture into a smooth paste, adding water as needed for desired consistency. In a separate small pan, heat the rest of the ½ tsp oil, and temper mustard seeds and urad dal. Pour this tempering over the chutney, and mix well. Serve the delicious horse gram chutney with idli, dosa or any other snack of your choice!

Lemon–Blueberry Oatmeal Cakes

Serves: 12
Preparation time: 15 minutes
Cooking time: 50 minutes

Ingredients
Old-fashioned rolled oats: 3 cups
Unsweetened almond milk/oat milk: 1¼ cups
Unsweetened applesauce: ½ cup
Maple syrup: ¼ cup
Lemon zest: 1 tbsp, grated
Lemon juice: ¼ cup
Eggs: 2 large
Baking powder: 1 tsp
Vanilla extract: 1 tsp
Salt: ¼ tsp

Frozen blueberries: 1 cup
Walnuts: 2 tbsp, chopped

Procedure

Set the oven to 375°F (190°C), and coat a muffin tin with cooking spray or line with silicone muffin liners. In a large bowl, combine rolled oats, almond milk, applesauce, maple syrup, lemon zest, lemon juice, eggs, baking powder, vanilla extract and salt. Stir well. Gently fold in the blueberries and chopped walnuts. Divide the mixture among the prepared muffin cups, about ⅓ cup each. Bake for 25 minutes or until a toothpick inserted into the centre comes out clean. Let the cakes cool in the pan for 10–15 minutes, then turn onto a wire rack. Serve warm or at room temperature.

The Learning

Eating for your heart doesn't mean sacrificing joy at the dining table. These recipes are proof that mindful choices can be delicious, satisfying and deeply nourishing. As you explore and experiment with these dishes, remember that every small step towards a heart-healthy lifestyle counts. So, savour each bite, embrace the goodness of whole foods and let your kitchen become the place where health and happiness go hand in hand. After all, the best way to care for your heart is to fill it – with love, laughter and, of course, great food.

More calcium in your bones = less calcium in your arteries. Weak bones (osteoporosis) often mean more calcium is deposited in your arteries, increasing heart risk.

29

Can Heart Diseases Be Reversed?

IMAGINE BEING TOLD THAT your heart, the very engine of your body, is wearing down – and that there's nothing you can do about it. For decades, heart disease was seen as an inevitable, progressive condition. But what if that is not entirely true? What if you could slow, halt or even partially reverse it? Science now suggests that with the right lifestyle changes, medications and medical interventions, it is possible to regain control over your heart health. The journey to a healthier heart isn't just about preventing further damage – it is about reclaiming vitality, energy and the promise of a longer, fuller life.

Yes, heart disease can be partially reversed, especially if detected early and treated aggressively with lifestyle changes, medication and sometimes medical procedures. While significant heart damage is hard to undo, steps can be taken to improve heart health, prevent progression and, in some cases, reduce plaque build-up in arteries.

Understanding Heart Disease and Reversibility

Heart disease often involves the build-up of plaque in the arteries, a condition called atherosclerosis. Over time, this can narrow the arteries, leading to restricted blood flow and increased heart attack or stroke risk. However, some evidence shows that with dedicated lifestyle changes, it is possible to reduce plaque build-up and improve blood flow, thus reducing risks.[1]

Lifestyle Changes as the Foundation

A heart-healthy lifestyle is essential for reversing heart disease. Here are key areas to focus on.

Diet

Eating a diet low in saturated fats, trans fats and cholesterol helps reduce plaque formation. The Mediterranean diet, rich in vegetables, fruits, whole grains, lean proteins and healthy fats like olive oil, has shown significant benefits. Limiting processed foods and added sugars is also critical.

Exercise

Regular physical activity strengthens the heart and improves circulation, helping to manage weight and lower blood pressure. Aerobic exercises like walking, swimming or cycling for 150 minutes a week are recommended. Over time, consistent exercise can improve blood vessel health and reduce artery stiffness.

Stress Management

Chronic stress raises cortisol levels, contributing to heart disease. Techniques like meditation, deep breathing exercises and yoga can help reduce stress. Reducing stress benefits heart health and can improve blood pressure and cholesterol levels.

Quit Smoking

Smoking accelerates plaque build-up and causes blood vessels to constrict. Quitting smoking is one of the best things you can do for heart health as it allows the body to start repairing itself.

Medical Management

Medications are often necessary to control factors contributing to heart disease. These include:

1. Statins: Statins lower LDL ('bad') cholesterol and have been shown to stabilise, or even reduce, plaque in arteries.

They are widely prescribed for heart disease prevention and reversal.
2. Blood pressure medications: High blood pressure is a major risk factor. Medications like ACE inhibitors, beta-blockers or calcium channel blockers help maintain healthy blood pressure and reduce strain on the heart.
3. Diabetes management: Proper control of blood sugar levels in diabetes patients is essential as high blood sugar contributes to atherosclerosis.

Advanced Therapies

In cases of severe atherosclerosis, procedures like angioplasty or coronary artery bypass surgery can restore blood flow to the heart muscle. These interventions don't cure heart disease but can relieve symptoms and reduce further damage.

Scientific Evidence of Reversal

Research has shown that intensive lifestyle changes, combined with medications, can reduce artery plaque. Studies by Dr Dean Ornish and others have found that a low-fat, plant-based diet, regular exercise, stress management and smoking cessation significantly improved heart disease markers.[2] Although plaque reduction may be modest, these changes improve overall heart function and reduce symptoms.

Reversing heart disease requires a comprehensive approach, combining lifestyle changes, medication and sometimes medical procedures. While damage may not be fully reversible, heart health can significantly improve, allowing individuals to lead longer, healthier lives.

The Learning

Heart disease doesn't have to be a one-way street. While reversing it completely may not always be possible, the power to slow its progression – and even improve heart function – is in your hands. With the right combination of diet, exercise, stress management and medical support, your heart can heal and strengthen over time. Every step you take towards a healthier lifestyle is a step towards a longer, more vibrant life. The question isn't just whether heart disease can be reversed – it is whether you're ready to take the first step.

> Some heart attacks can be reversed. If treated within the golden hour (first 60–90 minutes), damage can be minimised significantly.

30

Sudden Deaths in Young People

WHEN A YOUNG, SEEMINGLY healthy person dies suddenly, it is not only tragic but also puzzling for loved ones and the medical community. Such cases often reveal underlying conditions that are silent and undiagnosed, contributing to the growing awareness that sudden cardiac death isn't solely a risk for older individuals or those with known heart disease. Here's a look at the most common causes behind sudden deaths in young people without traditional risk factors.

Unseen Risks of Atherosclerosis and Beyond

The sudden death of a young person with no apparent risk factors is a tragic and shocking event. While traditionally considered a condition affecting older individuals with known cardiovascular risk factors, atherosclerosis has emerged as a significant underlying cause of sudden cardiac death even in seemingly healthy young people. Often, these young individuals may have underlying undiagnosed atherosclerosis with thin-cap fibroatheromas, vulnerable plaques prone to rupture, leading to fatal heart attacks.

The Role of Thin-Cap Fibroatheromas and Plaque Rupture

Atherosclerosis develops silently over years. In young individuals, thin-cap fibroatheromas are particularly dangerous. These plaques, with a thin fibrous cap overlying a lipid-rich core, are unstable and can rupture unexpectedly. When a rupture occurs, it triggers a cascade of blood clotting, leading to acute coronary occlusion – the sudden blockage of a coronary artery. This can halt blood flow to the heart, causing a fatal heart attack if not treated immediately. Unfortunately, in young individuals, this process often goes unnoticed until it is too late because it occurs without prior symptoms.

Diagnosing Vulnerable Plaques: Advanced Imaging Techniques

Standard diagnostic tools may not reveal the presence of thin-cap plaques, especially in younger people with no evident symptoms or traditional risk factors. However, advanced imaging techniques have improved our ability to identify high-risk plaques.

1. Optical coherence tomography: This high-resolution imaging modality allows us to visualise the thickness of the fibrous cap and assess plaque vulnerability. It can detect thin-cap fibroatheromas that may be at risk of rupture.
2. Lipid core burden index via near-infrared spectroscopy: This imaging technique measures the lipid content in coronary plaques. A high score indicates a lipid-rich, unstable plaque.
3. LipiScan: Another form of near-infrared spectroscopy technology, LipiScan provides real-time insights into the composition of coronary artery plaques, helping identify lipid-rich plaques that could lead to adverse events.

Non-Invasive Screening: Coronary CT Angiography and Calcium Scoring

For younger individuals without symptoms, non-invasive imaging can assess coronary health:

1. CT coronary angiography: This imaging provides detailed views of coronary anatomy and plaque characteristics,

making it possible to detect non-obstructive plaques that might otherwise go unnoticed.
2. Coronary calcium score: While not a direct measure of thin-cap fibroatheromas, this scan quantifies calcified plaques in the coronary arteries. Higher calcium scores indicate an elevated risk of atherosclerosis and future cardiovascular events.

Contributing Factors: Genetics, Stress and Inflammation

In some cases, young individuals may have hereditary risk factors for atherosclerosis, including elevated Lp(a) or familial hypercholesterolaemia, which predispose them to early plaque formation. Genetic screening and extended lipid profiles – including Lp(a) and apolipoprotein B levels – are valuable for identifying these risks.

Inflammation also plays a significant role. High-sensitivity C-reactive protein, an inflammatory marker, has been associated with an increased risk of plaque rupture and can identify those at higher risk despite normal cholesterol levels. Chronic stress, poor diet and environmental factors may further increase inflammatory markers, contributing to plaque instability.

Prevention and Awareness

The increasing incidence of sudden cardiac death in young individuals calls for greater awareness and preventive screening. Identifying hidden risks early, managing inflammation and monitoring lipid profiles – even in people without traditional risk factors – can help reduce this tragic occurrence. As we learn more about the role of thin-cap atherosclerosis, advanced imaging and tailored diagnostics offer new hope in catching silent threats before they lead to devastating outcomes.

From structural abnormalities to silent electrical disorders, understanding these underlying causes is crucial for awareness, early detection and prevention.

Cardiomyopathies: The Structural Culprits

1. HCM is one of the leading causes of sudden cardiac death in young people. This genetic condition causes the heart muscle, especially the left ventricle, to thicken abnormally, restricting blood flow and increasing the risk of arrhythmias. Often asymptomatic, HCM can go undetected until a sudden event occurs, such as during exercise when the heart is under stress.
2. Arrhythmogenic right ventricular cardiomyopathy is another inherited condition where fat and scar tissue replace parts of the right ventricular muscle, disrupting electrical signals and causing fatal arrhythmias. It often affects athletes, whose intense exercise can accelerate the disease.

Primary Electrical Disorders: The Silent Triggers

1. Long QT syndrome (LQTS) and Brugada syndrome are genetic disorders that affect the heart's electrical system. These conditions don't affect the heart's structure, so they often go undiagnosed, especially in young people. LQTS is characterised by a prolonged QT interval (a delay in the heart's electrical system's ability to recharge between beats, which can lead to life-threatening cardiac rhythms) on an ECG. This prolonged interval can lead to dangerous arrhythmias, especially during physical or emotional stress. Brugada syndrome, on the other hand, can cause sudden arrhythmias and is often responsible for unexpected nocturnal deaths.
2. Catecholaminergic polymorphic ventricular tachycardia (CPVT) is another rare genetic disorder where stress or exercise triggers rapid and irregular heartbeats that can result in fainting or sudden death.

Commotio Cordis: A Rare but Traumatic Cause

This phenomenon occurs when a young person receives a sudden, direct blow to the chest, often during sports. If the impact occurs at a specific point in the heart's electrical cycle, it can trigger a fatal arrhythmia. Although rare, commotio cordis underscores the importance of chest protection in contact sports.

Undiagnosed Congenital Heart Defects

Some young individuals may have been born with structural heart defects that went undetected due to a lack of symptoms. Conditions like anomalous coronary arteries, where the coronary arteries are abnormally placed, can impair blood flow to the heart muscle, particularly during exercise, leading to sudden cardiac arrest.

Substance Use and Stimulants

While young people without obvious risk factors may appear healthy, the use of substances like recreational drugs, certain prescription medications or even excessive energy drinks can overstimulate the heart, triggering arrhythmias or cardiac arrest. Cocaine, for instance, is a known trigger for sudden cardiac death, even in otherwise healthy individuals.

Myocarditis: The Inflammatory Threat

Inflammation of the heart muscle, often due to a viral infection, is known as myocarditis. Though rare, myocarditis can weaken the heart muscle and lead to arrhythmias. This risk has gained attention recently, especially with viral infections linked to myocarditis in younger populations.

The Learning

Sudden cardiac death in young people is often caused by hidden genetic or structural abnormalities, undetected congenital defects or external factors like trauma or substance use. While routine screening for these risks in all young people isn't currently feasible, heightened awareness and attention to warning signs — such as fainting during exercise, family history of sudden cardiac death or unexplained seizures — are crucial. Genetic testing, ECGs and other heart screenings for those with a family history or symptoms can sometimes uncover risks, providing an opportunity for preventive measures and potentially life-saving interventions.

> Sudden deaths in young people are often heart related. Undiagnosed hypertrophic cardiomyopathy, long QT syndrome or Brugada syndrome can cause cardiac arrest.

31

Palpitations

HAVE YOU EVER SUDDENLY felt your heart beating fast, skipping a beat, fluttering like a bird or pounding in your chest? Palpitations refer to the sensation of feeling your own heartbeat. This can be described as a rapid, irregular or forceful heartbeat. It can last for a few seconds or minutes and happen even when you're resting. Now, palpitations can happen for many reasons. Sometimes, they are harmless. Other times, they can be a sign of something more serious going on with your heart or body.

Supraventricular Tachycardia

In this condition, your heart suddenly starts beating very fast – sometimes between 150 and 250 beats per minute (normally, it is 60 to 100). This fast heartbeat starts from the top part of your heart, either in the upper chambers (called the atria) or in the part that connects the upper and lower parts (the AV node).

Symptoms can include palpitations, dizziness, shortness of breath, chest discomfort or even fainting in severe cases.

Is it lethal? It is usually not life-threatening but can be uncomfortable and alarming. It can sometimes require treatment to prevent recurrent episodes.

Ventricular Tachycardia

This is a rapid heart rate that originates in the ventricles. The heart rate is often over 100 beats per minute with potentially dangerous consequences.

Symptoms are similar to supraventricular tachycardia but can be more severe, including chest pain, shortness of breath, dizziness and loss of consciousness.

Is it lethal? Yes, ventricular tachycardia can be life-threatening, especially if it leads to ventricular fibrillation, which can cause sudden cardiac arrest if not treated immediately.

Causes of Palpitations

Palpitations can come from both heart-related (cardiac) and non-heart-related (non-cardiac) causes.

Cardiac Causes

These are more serious and should be checked by a doctor. They include:

1. arrhythmias (for example, supraventricular tachycardia, ventricular tachycardia, AFib)
2. heart disease (for example, CAD, heart failure)
3. valvular heart disease, and
4. cardiomyopathy (weak heart muscles)

Non-Cardiac Causes

1. Stress, anxiety or panic attacks
2. Excessive caffeine or alcohol consumption
3. Stimulant medications or recreational drugs
4. Hormonal changes (for example, during pregnancy, menopause or thyroid disorders)
5. Fever, dehydration or electrolyte imbalances
6. Anaemia

Understanding the cause of palpitations often requires a detailed medical history, physical examination and possibly tests like an ECG, Holter monitor or echocardiogram.

Atrial Fibrillation: The Most Common Irregular Rhythm

One of the most common causes of palpitations is atrial fibrillation or AFib.

What Is AFib?

AFib is when the top parts of your heart (the atria) beat in a very fast and messy way. Instead of contracting smoothly, they kind of shiver or flutter, which leads to a fast and irregular pulse. Your heart loses its usual rhythm, and the lower chambers (ventricles) also get irregular signals. It significantly increases the risk of stroke, heart failure and all-cause mortality. AFib can come and go on its own, last longer than a week or stay permanently depending on the type.

Types of AFib

1. Paroxysmal AFib comes and goes within seven days.
2. Persistent AFib lasts more than seven days or needs treatment to stop.
3. Permanent AFib is always there.

Features and Clinical Signs/Symptoms

AFib arises from ectopic foci, primarily in the pulmonary veins, leading to chaotic atrial electrical activity. The atrioventricular node transmits irregular impulses to the ventricles, causing an irregularly irregular rhythm.

Symptoms:

1. Palpitations (irregular and rapid heartbeat)
2. Fatigue and reduced exercise tolerance
3. Dyspnoea (shortness of breath)
4. Dizziness or syncope in severe cases
5. Chest discomfort or angina

In some cases, especially in older adults, AFib may be asymptomatic and diagnosed incidentally. Signs include:

1. irregularly irregular pulse,
2. variable intensity of heart sounds and
3. signs of heart failure, such as peripheral oedema or pulmonary rales, in advanced cases.

Diagnosis

1. Clinical evaluation: A detailed history and physical examination are critical to identify symptoms, triggers (for example, alcohol, stress) and underlying conditions (for example, hypertension, hyperthyroidism).
2. ECG reveals key findings such as an absence of P waves, the presence of irregular fibrillatory (f) waves and irregular RR intervals (the time interval between two consecutive R waves on the ECG tracing).
3. Advanced monitoring can be done with Holter monitoring or event recorders for paroxysmal AFib and implantable loop recorders for infrequent episodes.
4. Echocardiography evaluates left atrial size, left ventricular function and valvular abnormalities, while transoesophageal echocardiography can help spot any clots inside your heart.
5. Additional tests such as blood tests (for example, thyroid function, electrolytes, renal function) and chest X-ray and cardiac MRI in specific cases are done.

Latest Treatment Modalities

1. Rate control: The goal is to control the ventricular rate without necessarily restoring sinus rhythm. This doesn't fix the rhythm but slows down how fast the heart is beating. Doctors use beta-blockers (for example, metoprolol), non-dihydropyridine calcium channel blockers (for example, diltiazem, verapamil) and digoxin for rate control in heart failure patients.
2. Rhythm control: For symptomatic or recurrent AFib, restoring and maintaining sinus rhythm is

prioritised. Antiarrhythmic drugs such as Class III agents (amiodarone, dronedarone) and Class 1c agents (flecainide, propafenone) are administered.

3. Electrical cardioversion (electric shock) is effective in acute AFib.
4. Pharmacological cardioversion with agents like amiodarone or ibutilide is used.
5. Catheter ablation is a minimally invasive procedure where doctors insert thin tubes into your heart and use heat or cold energy to destroy the spots causing AFib. The most effective method is called pulmonary vein isolation.
6. Cryoablation or radiofrequency ablation techniques are commonly used.
7. Stroke prevention: AFib can cause blood to pool and form clots inside the heart. If a clot travels to the brain, it can cause a stroke. That is why preventing clots is so important in AFib patients.
    a. Oral anticoagulants (blood thinners): Non-vitamin K oral anticoagulants like dabigatran, rivaroxaban, apixaban, and edoxaban are preferred over warfarin for most patients.
    b. Warfarin is reserved for patients with mechanical valves or severe mitral stenosis.
    c. Left atrial appendage occlusion: Devices like the Watchman are options for patients at high bleeding risk who can't take blood thinners.
8. Lifestyle modification: Weight loss, exercise and management of risk factors like hypertension, diabetes and sleep apnoea are essential. AFib triggers (for example, alcohol, excessive caffeine) must be avoided.
9. Novel Treatments:
    a. Hybrid approaches such as combining catheter ablation and surgical techniques for persistent AFib

b. Use of genetics for precision medicine to understand which treatments will work best
   c. Electroporation ablation, a novel, non-thermal method showing promise in ongoing trials

The Learning

AFib is common but can be serious. It increases the risk of stroke and heart failure, but with the right care, people can live healthy, active lives. Thanks to modern treatments like new medications, advanced procedures and lifestyle changes, managing AFib has become much more effective.

The key is early diagnosis, a personalised treatment plan and regular follow-ups. Your heart may flutter – but your life doesn't have to.

> A racing heart isn't always due to anxiety. Frequent palpitations could be AFib or other arrhythmias, not just stress.

32

Breathing and Meditation

THE HEART, OFTEN REFERRED to as the engine of the body, plays a central role in maintaining life and health. Its continuous function ensures that oxygen and nutrients are delivered to tissues and organs throughout the body, while waste products are efficiently removed. However, the heart is not just influenced by physical activity, diet and medication; it is deeply affected by lifestyle factors, including rest, breathing and meditation. These often-overlooked factors are integral to maintaining heart health and preventing cardiovascular diseases.

This chapter delves into the intricate relationships between breathing and meditation and how each of these factors contributes to heart health. It also explores scientific findings, practical advice and ways to integrate these practices into daily life to ensure a healthy heart.

The Connection between Breathing and Heart Function

Breathing is a vital process that supports the exchange of gases in the lungs, ensuring that oxygen enters the bloodstream and carbon dioxide is expelled. While most people think of breathing as a simple, automatic action, it has a profound influence on heart health. Proper breathing techniques can help lower blood pressure, reduce anxiety and improve the efficiency of the cardiovascular system.

The rhythm of breathing is closely linked to heart rate through a phenomenon known as respiratory sinus arrhythmia, which refers to the natural variation in heart rate that occurs during the breathing cycle. When we inhale, the heart rate slightly increases, and when we exhale, it decreases. This natural fluctuation helps the heart work more efficiently and maintain optimal function.

How Breathing Affects Cardiovascular Function

Breathing has a direct impact on the autonomic nervous system, which regulates involuntary bodily functions like heart rate and blood pressure. Deep and slow breathing stimulates the parasympathetic nervous system, which calms the body and lowers heart rate. Conversely, rapid, shallow breathing or hyperventilation activates the sympathetic nervous system, leading to increased stress and heart rate.

Chronic stress can lead to sustained high levels of the stress hormone cortisol, which can increase blood pressure and lead to other heart disease risk factors. Practising controlled, slow breathing can counteract the effects of stress, leading to better cardiovascular health.

Breathing Techniques for Heart Health

The following breathing exercises are particularly beneficial for reducing stress, improving heart rate variability and supporting overall heart health.

Diaphragmatic Breathing

Also known as abdominal breathing, this technique involves inhaling deeply into the abdomen rather than shallowly into the chest. This activates the diaphragm and engages the parasympathetic nervous system, promoting relaxation.

How to Practise
Sit or lie down comfortably. Place one hand on your chest and the other on your abdomen. Breathe in slowly through your nose for a

count of 4, allowing your abdomen to rise. Exhale gently through your mouth for a count of 4. Repeat for 5–10 minutes.

Box Breathing

Box breathing is a technique used by the military and athletes to enhance focus and reduce stress. It involves equal-length inhales, holds and exhales.

How to Practise
Inhale for a count of 4, hold your breath for 4, exhale for 4 and hold again for 4. Repeat for several minutes.

Alternate Nostril Breathing (Nadi Shodhana)

This ancient yoga practice involves breathing through one nostril at a time, which is believed to balance the body's energy and promote calmness.

How to Practise
Sit comfortably, and close your right nostril with your thumb. Inhale deeply through your left nostril. Close your left nostril with your ring finger, and exhale through your right nostril. Inhale through your right nostril, then close it and exhale through your left nostril. Repeat the cycle for several minutes.

Meditation: A Path to Heart Health

Understanding the Benefits of Meditation

Meditation is a practice that involves focusing the mind and calming the body. It is often associated with mindfulness and relaxation but offers much more than just a moment of peace. Meditation has been shown to have profound benefits for heart health by reducing stress, lowering blood pressure and improving overall emotional well-being.

One of the primary ways meditation benefits the heart is by reducing stress. Stress is a well-known risk factor for heart disease, and chronic stress can lead to an increase in blood pressure, heart rate and inflammation, all of which contribute to cardiovascular problems. By practising mindfulness or relaxation techniques, individuals can break the cycle of stress and promote healing and balance within the body.

The Science Behind Meditation and Heart Health

Numerous studies have demonstrated the positive effects of meditation on cardiovascular health. For example, mindfulness meditation has been shown to lower blood pressure, reduce anxiety and improve heart rate variability, a key indicator of heart health. Meditation can also help reduce the risk of cardiovascular events such as heart attacks and strokes by lowering the levels of inflammatory markers and stress hormones in the body.

In addition to lowering stress, meditation enhances the vagus nerve, which is a key component of the parasympathetic nervous system. Activation of the vagus nerve helps lower heart rate and promotes relaxation, creating a more balanced and healthy heart function.

Meditation Practices for Heart Health

To integrate meditation into your daily routine, consider the following practices.

Mindfulness Meditation

This practice involves focusing on the present moment and accepting thoughts without judgement. It encourages awareness of breath, body sensations and emotions.

To practise it, sit comfortably with your eyes closed. Focus on your breath and observe how it enters and leaves your body. If your mind starts to wander, gently bring your attention back to your breath. Aim for 10–20 minutes per day.

Loving-Kindness Meditation (Metta)

This meditation focuses on cultivating compassion and kindness towards oneself and others, reducing negative emotions that can impact heart health.

To practise it, sit quietly, and focus on sending thoughts of love and compassion first to yourself, then to loved ones, acquaintances and even people you may have difficulties with. Silently repeat phrases like 'May I be happy, may I be healthy, may I be at ease'.

Transcendental Meditation

This practice involves repeating a mantra to help the mind reach a state of deep rest and alertness. Studies have shown that this practice can significantly lower blood pressure and reduce stress.[1]

To practise it, sit with your eyes closed, and silently repeat a mantra of your choosing for 15–20 minutes. It is best to practise twice a day.

The Learning

The importance of deep breathing and meditation in maintaining heart health cannot be overstated. These practices are not just ways to relax – they are vital components of a heart-healthy lifestyle. Proper sleep allows the heart to recover, while conscious breathing regulates stress and enhances cardiovascular function. Meditation offers a powerful tool for managing stress and improving overall well-being, directly benefiting the heart.

Incorporating these practices into daily life can lead to better emotional balance, reduced stress and a stronger, healthier heart. Whether through mindful breathing exercises, establishing a consistent sleep routine or engaging in meditation, these simple yet effective techniques can offer profound benefits for your cardiovascular system. By making sleep, breathing and meditation integral parts of your lifestyle, you can significantly reduce your risk of heart disease and improve your quality of life.

Ultimately, taking care of your heart isn't just about diet and exercise – it is about nurturing your mental and emotional health as well. With proper rest, deep breathing and meditation, you're not just protecting your heart; you're ensuring a longer, healthier and more fulfilling life.

> Heart attacks happen more often in the morning. Your body releases more stress hormones between 6 AM and 10 AM, making clots more likely to form.

33

Heart Health in Perimenopause and Menopause

HEART DISEASE IS THE leading cause of death for women worldwide, yet the risks associated with menopause and its impact on cardiovascular health often go unnoticed. Menopause marks a significant phase in a woman's life, typically occurring around the age of forty-five to fifty-five, characterised by the cessation of menstruation due to the decline of ovarian hormone production. This hormonal shift, particularly the drop in oestrogen levels, significantly affects cardiovascular health, increasing the risk of heart disease, hypertension and dyslipidaemia.

This chapter explores the connection between menopause and heart health, identifying risk factors, symptoms and preventive measures to empower women with the knowledge to safeguard their hearts during this transitional period.

Hormonal Changes and Heart Health

Oestrogen plays a vital role in protecting cardiovascular health.

1. Oestrogen helps to maintain healthy blood vessels. It supports the elasticity of blood vessels, aiding proper blood flow.
2. It regulates lipids. It promotes a favourable lipid profile, increasing HDL ('good' cholesterol) and reducing LDL ('bad' cholesterol).

3. Oestrogen has anti-inflammatory effects and reduces systemic inflammation, which is linked to atherosclerosis (plaque in arteries).

During perimenopause and menopause, declining oestrogen levels lead to:
1. loss of vascular elasticity (the blood vessels become stiff), increasing blood pressure;
2. changes in lipid metabolism, causing a rise in LDL and triglycerides while lowering HDL, and
3. heightened inflammation, exacerbating atherosclerosis and plaque formation.

These factors contribute to an increased risk of myocardial infarction, stroke and other cardiovascular diseases.

Risk Factors Unique to Menopause

While traditional cardiovascular risk factors – such as smoking, obesity and diabetes – remain relevant, menopause introduces additional concerns.
1. Weight gain and central obesity: Hormonal changes often lead to weight gain, especially around the abdomen, which is strongly associated with metabolic syndrome and insulin resistance.
2. Hypertension: Blood pressure tends to rise during menopause due to stiffening arteries and increased vascular resistance.
3. Dyslipidaemia: The lipid profile worsens during menopause, with higher LDL, lower HDL and elevated triglycerides, which accelerate atherosclerosis.
4. Insulin resistance and diabetes: Declining oestrogen levels may increase insulin resistance, raising the risk of type 2 diabetes – a significant cardiovascular risk factor.

5. Increased stress and anxiety: Hormonal fluctuations can exacerbate stress and depression, indirectly impacting heart health by encouraging unhealthy behaviours like poor diet and physical inactivity.

Symptoms of Heart Disease in Menopausal Women

Symptoms of cardiovascular disease in menopausal women may differ from those in men and are often subtle or overlooked. Common presentations include the following:

   1. Atypical chest pain (pressure or discomfort rather than sharp pain)
   2. Fatigue and shortness of breath (often mistaken for ageing or lack of fitness)
   3. Palpitations (resulting from hormonal changes or arrhythmias)
   4. Nausea and dizziness

Recognising these symptoms early is crucial for timely intervention.

Hormone Replacement Therapy and Heart Health

The role of hormone replacement therapy in cardiovascular health has been debated.

Benefits

   1. Improved lipid profile: Oestrogen can help reduce LDL and increase HDL levels.
   2. Vasodilation effects: Oestrogen may help maintain arterial flexibility.

Risks

   1. Increased thrombosis risk: Certain formulations of hormone replacement therapy can elevate the risk of deep vein thrombosis and pulmonary embolism.

2. Stroke: Higher doses of oestrogen, particularly in older women, may increase the risk of stroke.

Recommendations
1. Hormone replacement therapy is most beneficial when initiated early in menopause (within ten years of onset or before age sixty).
2. Individualised therapy is essential, weighing the benefits and risks for each woman.

Consultation with a healthcare provider is critical to determine the appropriate use of this therapy for cardiovascular protection.

Lifestyle Modifications for Heart Health

Lifestyle changes play a pivotal role in mitigating the cardiovascular risks associated with menopause.

Healthy Diet
1. Adopt a Mediterranean diet, rich in fruits, vegetables, whole grains, lean proteins and healthy fats, which supports heart health.
2. Reduce saturated fats and sugars by limiting processed foods, sugary beverages and high-fat snacks.
3. Include phytoestrogens by eating foods like soy, flaxseeds and legumes, which contain plant-based oestrogens that may help counterbalance hormonal decline.

Regular Exercise
1. Aim for 150 minutes of moderate aerobic exercise weekly, such as walking, cycling or swimming.
2. Incorporate strength training to maintain muscle mass and support metabolic health.
3. Yoga and Pilates can reduce stress and improve flexibility.

Weight Management

Maintaining a healthy weight reduces the risk of metabolic syndrome and its cardiovascular complications.

Stress Management

1. Practise mindfulness, meditation or deep breathing techniques.
2. Pursue hobbies, and maintain social connections to combat stress and anxiety.

Quit Smoking

Smoking accelerates vascular damage, and quitting significantly reduces cardiovascular risk.

Moderate Alcohol Consumption

Limit alcohol to one drink per day to avoid adverse effects on heart health.

Medical Screening and Monitoring

Regular health check-ups can help detect early signs of cardiovascular issues.

Recommended Screenings

1. Blood pressure monitoring: Aim for less than 120/80 mmHg.
2. Lipid profile: Check cholesterol levels at least once a year or more frequently if abnormal.
3. Blood sugar levels: Screen for diabetes through fasting glucose or HbA1c tests.
4. Weight and waist circumference: Monitor BMI and abdominal obesity.

Emerging Therapies and Interventions

1. Non-hormonal options: Medications like statins, ACE inhibitors or angiotensin receptor blockers (ARBs)

help manage cholesterol and blood pressure, offering alternatives to hormone replacement therapy for heart protection.
2. Sodium-glucose cotransporter 2 (SGLT2) inhibitors and glucagon-like peptide-1 (GLP-1) receptor agonists: Originally designed for diabetes, these drugs have shown cardiovascular benefits in reducing atherosclerosis (plaque build-up in arteries) and improving heart function.
3. Calcium and vitamin D supplementation: Preventing osteoporosis indirectly supports heart health by improving mobility and reducing stress-related risks.
4. Antioxidants: Supplements like omega-3 fatty acids and coenzyme Q10 may improve endothelial function and reduce inflammation.

Myths about Menopause and Heart Health

1. 'Heart disease is a man's problem': Women are equally at risk, especially post-menopause.
2. 'Symptoms of heart disease are the same for everyone': Women often experience atypical symptoms.
3. 'Hormone replacement therapy is always harmful': When used judiciously, it can benefit certain women.

Menopause, Mental Health and the Heart

The psychological effects of menopause – such as mood swings, depression and anxiety – can indirectly affect heart health by promoting unhealthy behaviours or increasing stress levels.

1. Cortisol: Chronic stress raises cortisol, contributing to hypertension and abdominal fat accumulation.
2. Sleep disturbances: Hormonal shifts disrupt sleep patterns, impairing heart health.

Addressing mental health is integral to a holistic approach to cardiovascular wellness.

When to Seek Medical Attention

Women experiencing the following should consult a healthcare provider immediately:

1. Persistent chest discomfort or pressure
2. Shortness of breath unrelated to exertion
3. Unexplained fatigue or palpitations
4. Symptoms of stroke, such as sudden weakness, confusion or facial drooping

The Learning

Menopause is a natural transition, but its impact on heart health demands attention. Women in perimenopause and menopause should prioritise preventive measures, including a heart-healthy lifestyle, regular screenings and personalised medical advice. By recognising symptoms early, addressing modifiable risk factors and staying informed, women can significantly reduce their cardiovascular risks and lead healthier, more fulfilling lives.

Heart health during menopause isn't just about managing symptoms – it is about taking proactive steps to safeguard long-term well-being.

> Heart disease can be silent for years. Diabetics, women and older adults may not feel chest pain even with severe heart disease.

34

Varicose Veins

VARICOSE VEINS ARE A common vascular condition that affects millions worldwide. Varicose veins are enlarged, twisted veins that often appear blue or purple. They usually occur in the legs and can be seen just under the skin. Advances in minimally invasive procedures like endovenous laser therapy (EVLT) have revolutionised the treatment landscape, offering effective alternatives to traditional surgical methods.

Understanding Varicose Veins Pathophysiology

The veins in the legs have trouble returning blood to the heart. This condition is often triggered by defective valves in the veins, which let blood flow backwards and pool instead of returning to the heart. These valves function like one-way doors, preventing backflow, but when they fail, blood accumulates, causing the veins to stretch and become varicose.

Who Is More Likely to Get Varicose Veins? (Risk Factors Explained Simply)

1. Age: Prevalence increases with age. The older you get, the more wear and tear your veins go through.
2. Gender: Varicose veins are more common in women due to hormonal influences (for example, pregnancy, menopause).
3. Genetics: Family history of varicose veins significantly raises risk.

4. Lifestyle factors: Prolonged standing or sedentary behaviour increases the risk. If you stand for long hours (like teachers, nurses or retail workers) or sit for too long without moving (like at a desk job), the blood has a harder time flowing back up your legs, increasing pressure in the veins.
5. Obesity: Extra weight increases venous pressure. Carrying extra body weight puts more pressure on your leg veins, making it harder for the blood to move upwards, and this adds strain on the valves.
6. Pregnancy: Increased blood volume and hormonal changes strain venous walls.

What Are the Symptoms?

1. Visible, bulging veins. You can see twisted, rope-like or bulging blue/purple veins on the legs
2. Leg heaviness, fatigue and discomfort
3. Swelling (oedema), particularly after standing for long periods
4. Skin changes, including hyperpigmentation and eczema. The skin around your ankles or calves might darken, itch or get dry and irritated. This happens when the poor blood flow starts affecting the skin
5. Ulceration in severe cases. In very serious cases, wounds or open sores can form near the affected area

Complications of Varicose Veins (What Can Go Wrong if Not Treated)

- Chronic venous insufficiency: Over time, if your veins continue to struggle with blood flow, it causes a condition called chronic venous insufficiency. This means your legs don't drain blood properly, which leads to long-term swelling (oedema) and damage to the skin – like thickening, discolouration or even scarring.
- Venous ulcers, typically around the ankles: When the skin and tissues are damaged for too long due to poor

circulation, painful wounds can develop near the ankles. These ulcers are slow to heal and often become a chronic issue.
- Thrombophlebitis (inflammation of a vein associated with clotting): Sometimes, blood clots can form inside a vein, causing it to become inflamed. This is called thrombophlebitis. It makes the vein painful, red and swollen – and it needs prompt medical attention.

Conservative Management

These are first-line treatments that don't involve surgery but help manage symptoms and prevent worsening.

1. Compression therapy: Compression stockings are special stockings that gently squeeze your legs, helping push blood back towards the heart. This reduces pressure in the veins and stops new varicose veins from forming. They're a go-to for everyday relief and prevention.
2. Lifestyle changes: Losing extra weight, staying active (like walking or doing leg exercises) and avoiding standing or sitting too long can ease symptoms. These habits reduce pressure on your leg veins and help with blood flow.
3. Medications: Venoactive drugs (for example, flavonoids) may help reduce leg heaviness and discomfort, but they won't fix the damaged veins. They're used for symptom management, not a cure.

Surgical Treatments

Here are some surgical options when first-line treatment does not work.

1. Vein stripping and ligation: This old-school method involves tying off and removing the damaged veins through incisions. While once the standard treatment, it is more invasive, comes with a longer recovery and has mostly been phased out in favour of newer techniques.

2. Phlebectomy: A less intense surgery where small varicose veins are removed through tiny cuts in the skin. It is often used for surface-level veins and has a shorter healing time.

Modern treatments are less painful, quicker to recover from and don't require hospitalisation. That is why the older methods are now reserved for rare cases.

EVLT: The Star of Modern Treatment

EVLT is a minimally invasive, outpatient procedure – meaning you walk in and walk out the same day.

Why It Is Preferred

There is less pain, no big cuts and a very short recovery time, and it is highly effective. It has become the go-to treatment for many patients with varicose veins.

Patient Selection

The treatment works best for people whose varicose veins cause symptoms like pain, heaviness or swelling – and where an ultrasound shows blood flowing in the wrong direction (reflux). If the veins are too twisted or curled (tortuous), it is hard to thread the laser through. Also, patients with certain serious circulation issues or blood clots in deep veins are not good candidates.

Ultrasound Mapping

A detailed ultrasound scan is done to create a 'map' of your leg veins, which helps the doctor see exactly which vein is malfunctioning. The scan also shows how bad the backflow is and how wide the vein is, which helps in planning the laser settings and treatment strategy.

Informed Consent

Before proceeding, the patient is given all the information – what the procedure involves, possible risks (like minor pain or bruising), benefits and expected results. Once everything is understood, the patient signs a consent form.

Steps of EVLT Procedure

Anaesthesia

Local tumescent anaesthesia, a special type of numbing medicine, is injected all around the vein. It has three jobs:

1. It numbs the area, so you don't feel pain.
2. It cools and protects the surrounding tissues from the laser heat.
3. It squeezes the vein slightly, which helps the laser work better.

Laser Fibre Insertion

1. A tiny incision is made in your skin. Using ultrasound (like a vein 'map'), a catheter is gently inserted into the problematic vein.
2. A hair-thin laser wire is then threaded through this tube and placed exactly where it needs to be – inside the affected vein.

Laser Energy Delivery

1. As the doctor slowly pulls the laser fibre out, the laser is turned on. It releases controlled heat directly onto the endothelium, the inner lining of the vein.
2. This heat damages the vein on purpose. So it shrinks, collapses and closes off completely – this is called fibrosis. Over time, the body naturally breaks down and absorbs this closed vein, and blood is naturally rerouted to healthier veins.

Post-Procedure Care

1. Right after the treatment, the patient will be made to wear tight-fitting stockings to help reduce swelling and bruises and support healing.

2. The patient is asked to walk around right after the procedure to keep the blood moving and lower the risk of blood clots.

Benefits of EVLT: Why Is It a Great Option?

1. Minimally invasive: The incision is so tiny that there's hardly any scar and a much lower chance of infection. It is performed under local anaesthesia – just a numbing shot. This makes the procedure safer and easier on your body.
2. High efficacy: The treatment works extremely well. Over 95 per cent of treated veins stay closed, and most people feel much better for a long time.
3. Quick recovery: Most patients return to normal activities within 24–48 hours with no long hospital stay or downtime.
4. Cosmetic advantage: Unlike old-fashioned surgery, EVLT doesn't leave big scars – your legs look better and feel better.

Complications of EVLT

While EVLT is considered very safe and effective, like any medical procedure, it can come with some risks. Here's what to be aware of:

1. Pain and bruising: Localised discomfort and bruising are common but resolve quickly.
2. Phlebitis: Sometimes the treated vein can get inflamed. This can be managed with anti-inflammatory medications.
3. Skin burns: Very rarely, if the laser fibre is too close to the skin or not properly placed, it can cause a burn on the skin above the vein. This is why ultrasound guidance and experienced hands are essential.
4. Nerve injury: Temporary numbness or tingling due to heat damage to nearby nerves may happen.

Varicose Veins

5. Deep vein thrombosis: This is the most serious, though extremely rare, risk. A blood clot could form in a deeper vein, which can be dangerous if not detected. That is why it is crucial to pick the right patients for EVLT and monitor them closely after the procedure (including encouraging walking and wearing compression stockings).

Comparison with Other Minimally Invasive Treatments

Radiofrequency Ablation

This method is similar to EVLT but uses radiofrequency energy instead of laser. It is slightly less painful post-procedure, but outcomes are comparable.

Sclerotherapy

This method uses a special chemical solution (sclerosant) injected directly into small veins to make them collapse and disappear. It is not a replacement for EVLT but is often used alongside it, especially for tiny leftover veins after the main ones are treated.

Mechanochemical Ablation

This newer technique uses a rotating wire to damage the vein's lining while also injecting the chemical solution, sclerosant, to close it off. Since it doesn't use heat like EVLT or radiofrequency ablation, it is less likely to cause skin burns or nerve issues, making it a gentle option for some patients.

Outcomes and Success Rates

Short-Term Results

1. Immediate symptom relief is observed in most patients. Most people feel better right after the procedure. The heaviness, aching and visible veins improve quickly.
2. In more than nine out of ten cases, the treated veins stay closed and stop causing trouble within a year.

Long-Term Outcomes

Once treated, most patients stay symptom-free. However, in some cases, symptoms can come back. Why? Two main reasons:

1. Even if old veins are closed, new problem veins can form later, especially if the underlying causes (like lifestyle or genetics) persist.
2. In rare instances, the treated vein might reopen, allowing blood to flow backwards again.
3. Getting periodic check-ups and making smart lifestyle choices, like staying active and maintaining a healthy weight, can help prevent recurrence.

Cost-Effectiveness of EVLT

EVLT might cost more upfront compared to things like compression stockings or medications, but it often saves money over time as there are fewer repeat problems, which means fewer future expenses. One-time laser treatment is often more lasting, so patients don't need multiple procedures. Since EVLT has a fast recovery time, people get back to work or life much sooner, saving time and income.

Future Directions in Varicose Vein Treatment

1. Advancements in laser technology: Newer lasers are being developed that use less intense heat, which may lower the risk of burns or nerve issues.
2. Combined modalities: Doctors are exploring using a mix of techniques (like EVLT with sclerotherapy) to treat all types and sizes of veins for better results.
3. Artificial intelligence (AI): AI tools can help doctors pinpoint problem veins more accurately and plan treatments with greater precision, improving outcomes.

The Learning

Varicose veins are not just a cosmetic concern but a significant medical condition that can impair quality of life. EVLT has emerged as a gold standard treatment, offering high efficacy, minimal invasiveness and excellent patient satisfaction. However, successful outcomes rely on proper patient selection, skilled operators and adherence to post-procedure care. As technology continues to evolve, EVLT and similar techniques promise even better results for patients suffering from varicose veins.

> 'Deep-vein thrombosis (DVT) poses a serious threat if the clot breaks off and travels to a blood vessel serving the lung, causing a potentially life-threatening blockage called a pulmonary embolism.'
>
> Lisa Catanese[1]

35

Valvular Heart Disease

YOUR HEART HAS FOUR valves that act like doors, ensuring blood flows in the right direction. Valvular heart disease occurs when these valves don't function properly, leading to issues like narrowing (stenosis) or leaking (regurgitation). Valvular heart disease is like a category of issues where the heart's valves don't work as they should.

The good news is that with better ways to detect and treat these valve problems – from high-tech heart scans to cutting-edge procedures – managing valvular heart disease today is more effective than ever. Patients now benefit from earlier diagnosis, more tailored treatments and faster recoveries, all of which contribute to longer, healthier lives.

This chapter delves into critical aspects of valvular diseases, focusing on balloon mitral valvotomy, prosthetic valves, non-rheumatic MR, tricuspid valve pathology and aortic stenosis.

Mitral Valve Disease

Mitral valve disease refers to any dysfunction of the valve between the heart's left chambers – either narrowing (stenosis), leaking (regurgitation) or both – that disrupts normal blood flow and strains the heart.

Balloon Mitral Valvotomy

This is a minimally invasive procedure (no big cuts or open-heart surgery needed!) that is done through the skin, usually through a vein in the leg. It is used to treat mitral stenosis, which is a condition where the mitral valve (the valve between the upper and lower left chambers of the heart) becomes too narrow. This narrowing is most often caused by old rheumatic fever, a disease that may have occurred years or even decades earlier.

When Do Doctors Consider Balloon Mitral Valvotomy?

Doctors consider this procedure when the patient has symptomatic severe mitral stenosis. The patient has clear symptoms (like breathlessness or fatigue), and tests show that the mitral valve opening is seriously narrowed – less than or equal to 1.5 cm^2 (a healthy valve is about 4-6 cm^2). The smaller the area, the harder it is for blood to flow, and the more pressure builds up in the lungs.

Before doing the valvotomy, doctors also check how 'pliable' or soft the valve is. They use something called the Wilkins score, which rates how thick, stiff or calcified the valve and surrounding tissues are. A score of 8 or less means the valve is still soft enough to respond well to balloon treatment. If the valve is too calcified or damaged, balloon mitral valvotomy might not work.

Procedure

1. A catheter is gently threaded up to the heart through a vein in your leg.
2. At the tip of this catheter is a special balloon. Once it reaches the narrow mitral valve, the balloon is inflated right inside it.
3. This inflation forces the stuck parts of the valve (called commissures) to separate, creating a wider opening.

That means better blood flow and less pressure on the lungs.

Outcomes

1. The effect is usually instant: the valve opens up more (mitral valve area increases), which improves how blood

flows through the heart. This is what doctors call a 'haemodynamic improvement'.
2. Patients often feel better quickly – less breathlessness, more energy – because the lungs don't have to deal with so much backed-up pressure anymore. It is like taking a weight off your chest.

Limitations
1. If the valve is leaking badly (MR) or is too stiff and calcified, this procedure is not an option. In such cases, other treatments like surgery might be safer.
2. While balloon mitral valvotomy is generally safe, it is still a procedure inside your heart. So it carries some risk. Rarely, bits of clot or debris can break off and cause an embolism (a blockage somewhere else in the body), or the balloon could tear the valve (perforation), leading to serious problems that might need urgent surgery.

Prosthetic Mitral Valve

When a patient's mitral valve is too damaged for a balloon procedure or keeps getting blocked or leaky, the best option is to replace it with an artificial valve.

Types of Prosthetic Valves

Mechanical Valves

Mechanical valves are built to last a lifetime, but the patient must take blood thinners every day to prevent clots from forming on the valve.

Bioprosthetic Valves

Bioprosthetic valves, often made from animal tissue, don't last as long (usually around ten to fifteen years), but they're gentler on the body as there is no need for daily blood thinners. Hence, they're often chosen for older patients who may not tolerate long-term medication well.

Key Considerations

Blood Thinners Are a Must (for Mechanical Valves)

If a patient gets a mechanical valve, they'll need to take a blood thinner like warfarin for life. The goal is to keep the blood's clotting ability within a safe range – known as the international normalised ratio – ideally between 2.5 and 3.5, to avoid dangerous clots on the valve.

Valve Lifespan

Mechanical valves last twenty to thirty years, while bioprosthetic valves typically last ten to fifteen years.

Possible Complications

1. Blood clots (thrombosis) or excess tissue growth (pannus) can block the valve and make it malfunction. Both are serious and need quick medical attention.
2. Just like natural valves, artificial ones can get infected, a serious condition called endocarditis, which can damage the valve and lead to major complications.

Non-Rheumatic MR

While rheumatic fever is a common cause of MR, many cases today are non-rheumatic. It could happen due to wear and tear, damage from a heart attack or changes in the size and shape of the heart. In non-rheumatic MR, structural abnormalities of the mitral valve, such as prolapse, flail leaflets or annular dilation, contribute to regurgitation.

What Causes Non-Rheumatic MR?

Degenerative MR

It could be age-related 'wear and tear' of the mitral valve. The valve becomes floppy (called mitral valve prolapse) because its tissue weakens – a bit like a stretched-out elastic.

Sometimes, the supporting strings (called chordae) can snap, causing part of the valve to swing wildly. This is known as a flail leaflet.

Ischaemic MR

After a heart attack, the muscles that hold the valve steady (papillary muscles) can get damaged or die. This makes the valve less effective at closing tightly.

Functional MR

Here, the valve itself is fine, but the problem lies in the left ventricle (the main pumping chamber). If the ventricle stretches out or weakens, the valve can't close properly. This is common in dilated cardiomyopathy.

Diagnosis

1. Echocardiography is the gold standard for assessing MR. It uses sound waves to create images of your heart and shows how badly the valve is leaking.
2. Transoesophageal echocardiography is a more detailed version of echo.

Managing MR: From Medicines to Modern Interventions

Treating MR is all about easing symptoms, preventing heart failure and fixing the leaky valve when necessary. The approach depends on the cause and severity of MR and the patient's overall health.

Medical Therapy: Support, Not a Cure

1. Diuretics help get rid of excess fluid, easing breathlessness and swelling.
2. ACE inhibitors or ARBs reduce the pressure against which the heart pumps (afterload), which is especially

helpful in functional MR where the problem lies more in the ventricle than the valve itself.

Note: Medicines don't fix the valve – they just buy time or help control symptoms.

When Medicine Isn't Enough: Repair or Replace
1. Mitral valve repair is the gold standard for degenerative MR. It keeps the native valve intact, preserving natural heart function. It is ideal when the valve is structurally repairable.
2. Mitral valve replacement is used when repair isn't possible and the valve is too damaged. The diseased valve is removed and replaced with a mechanical or bioprosthetic valve.

MitraClip: For Those Who Can't Have Surgery

A transcatheter is a non-surgical and minimally invasive option where a clip is delivered through a vein. It is ideal for high-risk patients who can't tolerate open-heart surgery.

Tricuspid Valve Disease

Tricuspid valve disease refers to any disorder affecting the tricuspid valve, which controls blood flow between the right atrium and right ventricle of the heart. It most commonly presents as TR – where the valve doesn't close properly, causing blood to leak backwards.

Causes

Tricuspid valve disease, particularly TR, is frequently a result of underlying diseases rather than a valve-specific issue. Two significant causes are left heart disease and pulmonary hypertension. Primary causes may be infection, congenital defects or tumours. Though often overlooked, it plays a crucial role in overall heart function and is gaining attention in modern cardiology.

Diagnosis

1. Echocardiography measures the leak and looks at right heart function.
2. MRI or CT are useful if anatomy is complex or other structures need better visualisation.

Management: Fixing the Leak

1. Medical therapy: Diuretics help reduce fluid overload (swelling, liver congestion and so on), but again, like MR, this is symptom control – not a cure.
2. Surgical interventions:
    a. Repair (annuloplasty) is preferred in functional TR. This procedure tightens the ring of the valve.
    b. Replacement is reserved for very severe cases or when repair isn't possible.
3. Transcatheter interventions: Emerging therapies like TriClip provide novel therapeutic alternatives for high-risk patients.[1]

Aortic Valve Disease

Aortic valve disease, especially aortic stenosis, is a major concern in older adults. It occurs when the aortic valve narrows, making it harder for blood to exit the heart, which puts strain on the left ventricle.

Aetiology (Causes)

1. Degenerative aortic stenosis is the most common – calcium builds up on the valve with age.
2. Rheumatic aortic stenosis is now rare. It is linked to past rheumatic fever, causing valve fusion.

Pathophysiology

As the valve narrows, the heart has to work harder to push blood through, leading to thickening of the heart muscle (left ventricle hypertrophy), reduced relaxation (diastolic dysfunction) and, ultimately, heart failure.

Symptoms
1. Shortness of breath (dyspnoea)
2. Chest pain (angina)
3. Fainting spells (syncope)
4. Heart failure in advanced stages

Diagnosis
Echocardiography is the go-to test. It evaluates:
1. aortic valve area (severe if less than 1 cm^2),
2. pressure gradients (severe if greater than or equal to 40 mmHg) and
3. CT calcium score (helpful when echo results are ambiguous, especially in low-gradient aortic stenosis).

Management
1. Medical therapy plays a limited role and focuses on symptom control.
2. Surgical aortic valve replacement is the gold standard for symptomatic aortic stenosis in low-risk patients.
3. TAVR is a minimally invasive option for high-risk surgical candidates.

Challenges in Combined Valvular Pathology

When a patient has more than one valve affected – like TR, aortic stenosis and MR – treatment becomes far more complex.

1. Haemodynamic complexity: The heart's right and left sides influence each other. Fixing one valve can unmask or worsen another issue, so everything must be evaluated as a system, not in isolation.

2. Surgical risk: Operating on multiple valves means longer procedures, higher chances of complications and tougher recovery – especially in older or frail patients.
3. Timing of intervention: Deciding when to intervene depends on a mix of factors: how bad the symptoms are, how well the heart is pumping and whether the patient has other health issues. Delaying too long risks heart failure; acting too soon may expose them to unnecessary risk.

Future Perspectives

Advances in transcatheter therapies, such as TAVR, MitraClip and TriClip, continue to expand the treatment landscape, offering options for patients previously deemed inoperable. Additionally, innovations in imaging and biomarker research promise earlier detection and personalised treatment strategies for valvular heart disease.

The Learning

Valvular heart disease spans a broad spectrum of conditions, each demanding accurate diagnosis and individualised treatment strategies. With the evolution of surgical and transcatheter techniques – and the power of collaborative, multidisciplinary care – patient outcomes have significantly improved. Yet, as the field continues to evolve, ongoing innovation and research are essential to overcome existing challenges and meet the needs of an increasingly complex patient population.

> A 'normal' ECG doesn't rule out a heart problem. An ECG can be normal even if you have a heart blockage, especially if it is early or intermittent.

36

Mending the Holes in the Heart: Device Closure Versus Surgery

HOLES IN THE HEART, medically known as septal defects, are a significant source of concern for parents, carers and individuals diagnosed with such conditions. While the phrase 'hole in the heart' can sound alarming, many of these defects are benign and manageable with modern medical care. This chapter aims to demystify the topic, explain how these conditions are identified and treated, and provide clarity on what to do if a defect is discovered.

What Are Holes in the Heart?

The heart is divided into four chambers: two upper atria and two lower ventricles. These chambers are separated by thin walls called septa. The atrial septum separates the left and right atria. The ventricular septum separates the left and right ventricles.

A 'hole in the heart' occurs when there is a defect in one of these septa, allowing blood to flow abnormally between the chambers. These defects can be congenital (present at birth) or acquired (develop later in life due to infections or trauma).

Types of Holes in the Heart

1. ASD: ASD is when there is a hole in the wall between the two atria. In this condition, the oxygen-rich blood from the left atrium mixes with oxygen-poor blood in the right atrium.

2. VSD: VSD is when there is a hole in the wall between the two ventricles. It causes the oxygen-rich blood from the left ventricle to flow into the right ventricle, leading to inefficient oxygen delivery.
3. Patent foramen ovale (PFO): In this condition, a small, flap-like opening between the atria fails to close after birth. This is often asymptomatic and considered benign unless associated with complications like strokes.
4. Complete atrioventricular septal defect: A larger defect affecting both atrial and ventricular septa, this defect is common in conditions like Down syndrome.
5. Acquired defects: They are usually rare but can occur due to trauma or infections (for example, infective endocarditis) or after a heart attack.

How Are These Defects Identified?

Holes in the heart may not always produce symptoms, especially if they are small. However, certain signs or diagnostic techniques can help identify them.

Symptoms

If the defects are small, they are often asymptomatic. But if the defects are large, they may cause the following:

1. Fatigue during exercise
2. Shortness of breath
3. Frequent lung infections
4. Poor growth and feeding difficulties in children
5. Cyanosis in severe cases

Physical Examination

Doctors may hear a murmur (an abnormal heart sound) during a routine check-up, prompting further evaluation.

Diagnostic Tests

1. Echocardiography is the primary tool to visualise heart structure and blood flow.
2. Transoesophageal echocardiography provides detailed images in certain cases.
3. Cardiac MRI or CT scans help assess complex defects.
4. Chest X-rays can reveal an enlarged heart or increased blood flow to the lungs.
5. ECGs detect electrical activity changes due to septal defects.
6. Cardiac catheterisation measures pressures and oxygen levels in the chambers to confirm the diagnosis.

What Happens if a Hole Is Found?

When a septal defect is detected, the next steps depend on its size, location and impact on heart function. Here's what typically happens.

Watchful Waiting

Small defects (ASD, VSD, PFO) often close on their own during childhood. These cases may not require treatment but are monitored periodically with echocardiograms.

Medical Management

The following medications may be prescribed to manage symptoms or complications:

1. Diuretics to reduce fluid build-up in the lungs
2. ACE inhibitors or beta-blockers to help manage heart failure in symptomatic patients
3. Anticoagulants to prevent clot formation in PFO-related strokes

Intervention for Larger Defects

1. Catheter-based closure is a minimally invasive procedure where a closure device is inserted through a

catheter to seal the defect. It is common for ASDs and some VSDs.
2. Surgical repair through open-heart surgery may be required for larger or more complex defects (for example, atrioventricular septal defect). It involves sutures or a patch to close the hole.

Treatment of Acquired Defects

The underlying cause (for example, infections, trauma) must be addressed.

What Happens After Closure?

Whether the hole closes naturally, through a device or via surgery, long-term outcomes are usually excellent. However, follow-up care is crucial.

1. Regular check-ups: Heart function should be monitored, particularly in childhood and adolescence.
2. Activity restrictions: Most children and adults can lead normal, active lives. Extreme activities may require clearance in certain cases.
3. Infective endocarditis prophylaxis: This means taking preventive measures (usually in the form of antibiotics). Antibiotics may be needed before dental or surgical procedures to prevent infection in certain cases.

Complications if Left Untreated

Large or untreated holes can lead to complications:

1. Heart failure due to overloading of the heart
2. Pulmonary hypertension
3. Arrhythmias
4. Eisenmenger syndrome
5. Stroke (blood clots can pass through a PFO or ASD and cause a stroke)

What Should Parents or Patients Do?

If you or your child is diagnosed with a hole in the heart, here's a step-by-step approach:

1. Stay calm: Most defects are manageable, and many close on their own. Seek detailed guidance from a cardiologist.
2. Seek expert opinion: Paediatric cardiologists specialise in congenital heart defects, while adult cardiologists handle acquired or residual issues.
3. Follow up regularly: Keep up with scheduled echocardiograms and other tests.
4. Promote a healthy lifestyle: Ensure good nutrition and adequate exercise, and avoid smoking or second-hand smoke exposure.
5. Recognise symptoms early: Know the warning signs of complications like fatigue, cyanosis (bluish discolouration of the skin, lips or nail beds, which is a visible sign that there is not enough oxygen in the blood) or difficulty breathing.

Advantages of Device Closure

1. No visible scars or stitches: The device closure is performed through a small puncture in the groin, leaving no chest scars.
2. Avoidance of general anaesthesia: Many of these procedures can be done with sedation rather than full anaesthesia.
3. Faster recovery: Since device closures are minimally invasive, patients usually recover more quickly and can resume normal activities sooner.

When Intracardiac Repair Is Needed

1. Inadequate margins: If the edges around the defect are not strong or large enough to hold a device securely, surgical repair is necessary.

2. Large or complex defects: Defects that are too large or involve multiple areas, as seen in some atrioventricular septal defects and large VSDs, often require open-heart surgery.
3. Associated valve abnormalities: In cases where the defect affects surrounding valves, surgical repair allows for comprehensive treatment of both the defect and any valve issues.

Common Questions about Holes in the Heart

1. Will the Hole Close on Its Own?
Small ASDs and VSDs often close naturally by the age of five. Larger defects typically require intervention.

2. Are All Holes Dangerous?
Many small defects are harmless, but larger ones may need treatment to prevent complications.

3. Can Adults Have Undiagnosed Holes?
Yes, some defects like PFOs remain undiagnosed until adulthood, often after a stroke or unexplained symptoms.

4. How Is a Hole Closed Without Surgery?
Catheter-based closure involves threading a device through a vein to seal the hole, avoiding open-heart surgery.

Advancements in Treatment

The management of septal defects has come a long way with minimally invasive techniques, advanced imaging and personalised care. Innovations like 3D echocardiography, robot-assisted surgery and biodegradable closure devices continue to improve outcomes.

The Learning

'Holes in the heart' might sound frightening, but with early detection, appropriate management and regular follow-up, most patients can live healthy, normal lives. If you suspect or know of a septal defect in yourself or your child, consult a cardiologist promptly.

Stay informed, follow medical advice and maintain a healthy lifestyle for the best outcomes.

For many types of congenital heart defects, especially small to moderate holes, treatment has advanced to include minimally invasive device closures that avoid the need for traditional surgery. This approach is preferred when possible as it eliminates the need for scars, stitches and general anaesthesia, provided that the structural margins around the defect are suitable. If the margins are insufficient or the defect is too large, traditional intracardiac repair through open-heart surgery may be necessary.

> 'Demographic data indicate that the heart disease rate among Indians is double that of national averages of the Western world.'
>
> Indian Heart Association[1]

37

Chest Pain

CHEST PAIN IS ONE of the most common complaints in ERs worldwide. While a normal ECG can often reassure patients and physicians alike, it does not rule out potentially life-threatening conditions such as acute coronary syndrome. A systematic approach is essential to determine the underlying cause, ensuring prompt and accurate diagnosis while avoiding unnecessary risks.

This discussion will look at three important things in managing heart-related issues:

1. The role of cardiac biomarkers: These are substances in the blood that can indicate how well the heart is functioning or if it is damaged. Doctors test for these markers to help diagnose heart problems.
2. Strain-rate echocardiography: This is a special type of ultrasound that helps doctors see how well the heart is pumping. It measures how the heart muscle is stretching and contracting, which gives important information about heart health.
3. Patient observation: This means closely monitoring the patient to watch for any changes in their condition. By keeping track of symptoms and overall health, doctors can make better decisions about treatment.

Combining these tools helps doctors effectively care for patients with heart issues.

An initial assessment is done to prioritise high-risk features.

Importance of History and Physical Examination

Before making any decisions about a patient's heart condition, it is vital to gather detailed information. Key factors to consider include the following:

- Nature of pain: Understand the type of pain (sharp, dull), its duration, where it is located and if it spreads to other areas.
- Associated symptoms: Look for other symptoms like difficulty breathing (dyspnoea), sweating (diaphoresis), rapid heartbeat (palpitations), nausea or fainting (syncope).
- Risk factors: Consider if the patient smokes or has high blood pressure (hypertension), diabetes, high cholesterol (dyslipidaemia), a family history of heart disease or previous heart issues.

A focused physical exam can also provide helpful clues. For example, low blood pressure (hypotension), fast heartbeat (tachycardia) or signs of heart failure might suggest serious heart problems like reduced blood flow (ischaemia).

Role of ECG

While a normal ECG can be reassuring, it is important to remember its limitations.

1. Sensitivity: It only detects acute ischaemia about half the time (50 per cent).
2. Detection gaps: It might miss ischaemia in some cases:
   a. Myocardial infarction at the back of the heart (posterior)
   b. Problems with the right side of the heart (isolated right ventricular infarction)
   c. Small blood vessel issues (microvascular angina)
   d. Early stages of certain heart attacks, such as non-ST elevation myocardial infarction (NSTEMI)[1]

Performing serial ECGs during chest pain can show dynamic changes that suggest ischaemia.

Cardiac Biomarkers: Finding Subtle Myocardial Injury (Heart Damage)

High-Sensitivity Troponin (hs-Tn)

Troponin is a key marker for diagnosing acute coronary syndrome. Its benefits include high sensitivity as it effectively detects heart damage and early detection as it can find minor heart damage that other tests might miss.

By taking measurements at the start and again after 3 hours, doctors can see if levels are changing:

1. Rule-in criteria: There is significant increase or decrease in troponin levels alongside clinical symptoms.
2. Rule-out criteria: Troponin levels remain below the 99th percentile and stable over time.

Other Biomarkers

While troponin remains the gold standard, other markers such as creatine kinase-MB (CK-MB; the MB refers to the two protein subunits, M and B, that make up this particular form of the enzyme) and myoglobin are less specific and rarely used in modern practice. Emerging markers such as high-sensitivity C-reactive protein (hs-CRP) and brain natriuretic peptide (BNP) may assist in specific scenarios.

Strain-Rate Echocardiography: An Advanced Imaging Method

Principles of Strain-Rate Echocardiography

Strain-rate imaging looks at how heart tissue changes shape abnormally (myocardial deformation), giving information on subtle heart problems that regular echocardiograms might miss.

Benefits

Strain-rate imaging can identify movement issues in the heart caused by reduced blood flow. Also, it measures heart muscle efficiency even when there are no obvious motion problems.

Application in Chest Pain

A normal strain pattern strongly suggests that there is no significant heart problem. Abnormal strain values can help pinpoint areas of reduced blood flow before other tests show harm. Global longitudinal strain (GLS) helps distinguish between reduced blood flow and other chest pain causes, such as inflammation of the heart muscle (myocarditis).

Observation and Monitoring

For patients with chest pain but a normal ECG, close monitoring is still necessary, especially if there are high-risk features or diagnostic uncertainty.

Establishing a Chest Pain Unit (CPU) Protocol

By observing patients in a CPU, healthcare teams can provide structured care and conduct repeat tests:
1. Repeat ECGs every 15–30 minutes or during episodes of pain
2. Serial troponin measurements at 0, 3 and 6 hours after arrival
3. Echocardiography within 24 hours to check for motion problems in the heart walls

Clinical Scoring Systems

Tools like the HEART score help assess risk and direct treatment:
1. Components: Evaluate history, ECG, age, risk factors and troponin levels.
2. Scoring: A score of 3 or less means low risk; 7 or higher indicates high risk, possibly needing admission or invasive actions.

Diagnostic Approach

Low-Risk Patients

1. Consider discharging after negative troponin and normal ECGs if no concerning symptoms arise.
2. Schedule functional tests (for example, stress echo or MRI) as needed.

Intermediate-Risk Patients

1. Recommend advanced imaging like strain-rate echo, coronary CT angiography or stress tests.
2. Some may require longer observation or admission if results are unclear.

High-Risk Patients

Immediate cardiology consultation is necessary for more invasive tests or urgent treatments.

Common Non-Cardiac Causes of Chest Pain

Gastrointestinal Issues

Conditions like gastro-oesophageal reflux disease, oesophageal spasms or peptic ulcers can feel like heart pain. Doctors may use antacids or a test called oesophagogastroduodenoscopy to help diagnose these issues.

Pulmonary Problems

Lung conditions such as pulmonary embolism, pneumothorax (collapsed lung) or pleuritis (inflammation of the lung lining) can also cause chest pain. Tests like D-dimer testing and CT pulmonary angiography can help rule out pulmonary embolism.

Musculoskeletal Causes

Pain from conditions like costochondritis (inflammation of the rib cartilage) or muscle strain is often tender to the touch and can mimic heart pain.

Psychogenic Factors

Anxiety or panic attacks can cause chest pain, but it is important to rule out other possible causes first.

Special Considerations

Women and Atypical Presentations

Women may experience atypical symptoms such as fatigue or indigestion instead of classic chest pain. A condition called myocardial infarction with non-obstructive coronary arteries happens more often in women and might require special imaging to diagnose.

Young Adults and Athletes

In these individuals, consider conditions like myocarditis (inflammation of the heart), abnormalities in coronary arteries or spontaneous coronary artery dissection.

Older Adults with Comorbidities

Older patients may experience silent ischaemia (lack of blood flow with no obvious symptoms) or unusual symptoms, making it crucial to be vigilant.

Treatment Principles

Acute Management

1. Administer aspirin unless there's a reason not to.
2. Nitroglycerin can help relieve chest pain caused by decreased blood flow, but it must be used carefully in patients with low blood pressure.

Secondary Prevention

If ischaemia is confirmed, start treatments like statins, ACE inhibitors or beta-blockers.

Non-Ischaemic Chest Pain

Treatment should be tailored based on the specific cause of the pain.

Limitations of Current Tools

Troponin

Elevated troponin levels can occur in conditions that do not involve ischaemia, such as myocarditis or sepsis. Troponin tests may not be sensitive enough in the early stages of heart injury.

ECG

An ECG may appear normal even in the early stages of ischaemia or certain patterns of heart attacks.

Strain-Rate Echo

This test can be limited by availability and the skills of the person conducting it.

The Learning

Experiencing chest pain with a normal ECG is common and can be tricky to evaluate in the ER. A carefully planned approach that includes thorough clinical evaluation, repeated tests for heart-related markers and advanced imaging techniques like strain-rate echocardiography is important to identify serious conditions and avoid unnecessary procedures. Observing patients in a specialised CPU, guided by risk assessment tools like the HEART score, helps ensure safe and effective care. Quick and informed decision-making can greatly influence patient outcomes, highlighting the value of combining clinical expertise with proven medical practices.

> Heart attacks don't always cause chest pain. Many people experience symptoms like jaw pain, nausea, sweating or breathlessness instead.

38

Coronary Artery Bypass Surgery

CORONARY ARTERY BYPASS GRAFTING (CABG) is a life-saving surgery for patients with severe CAD. The success of this procedure largely depends on how long the grafts used in surgery remain open and functional. The most commonly used vein for this is the saphenous vein, but these vein grafts have a tendency to become blocked over time. This chapter explains how long vein grafts last, why they get blocked and how medications like antiplatelets and statins help improve their lifespan.

Lifespan of Vein Grafts: How Long Do They Last?

Phases of Vein Graft Failure

After being implanted, vein grafts undergo changes that can eventually lead to blockage. This failure happens in three stages:

Early Graft Failure (Within One Month)

Around 12 to 20 per cent of vein grafts fail in the first month because blood clots form due to surgical issues, poor blood flow or damage to the vein's inner lining.

Intermediate Graft Failure (One Month to One Year)

Around 15 to 25 per cent of vein grafts fail during this time because the vein thickens due to smooth muscle cell growth, narrowing the blood vessel.

Late Graft Failure (After One Year)

Within ten years, 50 per cent of vein grafts fail because of progressive hardening and narrowing of the vein due to fatty deposits and inflammation.

Comparing Vein Grafts and Arterial Grafts

Arterial grafts (for example, internal mammary arteries) have a 90 per cent success rate after ten years because they are more resistant to blockages.

Vein grafts are easier to harvest but have a 50 per cent success rate at ten years, requiring more monitoring and preventive care.

Why Do Vein Grafts Get Blocked?

Surgical Factors

1. Damage during graft removal or placement can cause clot formation.
2. Poor surgical connections can create turbulent blood flow, increasing clot risk.

Patient-Related Factors

1. Uncontrolled risk factors: High blood pressure, diabetes, smoking and high cholesterol speed up graft blockages.
2. Blood clotting disorders: Conditions like AFib or inherited blood disorders increase the risk of clotting in grafts.

Vein Graft Characteristics

1. Unlike arteries, veins lack a strong elastic layer, making them more vulnerable to structural changes under high-pressure arterial blood flow.
2. If the coronary artery being bypassed is very narrow, the graft may not receive enough blood flow to stay open.

How Medications Improve Vein Graft Longevity

Antiplatelet Therapy

This therapy is needed to prevent clots in grafts. Injury during graft harvesting damages the vein's lining, increasing the risk of clot formation.

Recommended Medications

1. Dual antiplatelet therapy: Aspirin and a P2Y12 inhibitor (clopidogrel) should be taken for at least twelve months after surgery to prevent early failure.
2. Single antiplatelet therapy: After one year, most patients continue aspirin for life to prevent long-term graft closure.
3. For aspirin-allergic patients: Clopidogrel is an alternative.

The PREVENT IV trial found that strong blood-thinning therapy reduces early graft failure.[1]

Statins (Preventing Graft Narrowing and Hardening)

Statins are important because they lower cholesterol and stabilise blood vessels, preventing fatty build-up in grafts.

Recommended Medications

1. High-intensity statins (for example, atorvastatin 40–80 mg/day) for all CABG patients, regardless of cholesterol levels
2. Target LDL cholesterol should be below 55 mg/dL for high-risk patients

Lifelong use is necessary to keep grafts open.

The RESEARCH registry shows that patients on statins had 40 per cent less graft narrowing over ten years.[2]

Additional Medications to Support Graft Health

1. Beta-blockers to reduce heart strain and improve heart function after CABG
2. ACE inhibitors/ARBs to protect blood vessels, especially in patients with high blood pressure or diabetes
3. Ezetimibe and PCSK9 Inhibitors to lower cholesterol further if statins alone are not enough

Long-Term Prevention Strategies

Lifestyle Changes

1. Quit smoking (the most important step).
2. Exercise regularly as it helps maintain heart and vessel health.
3. Follow a healthy diet such as the Mediterranean diet (rich in vegetables, fish and healthy fats), which reduces cholesterol and inflammation.

Managing Health Conditions

1. Diabetes: Keeping blood sugar levels under control prevents small blood vessel damage.
2. High blood pressure: Keeping blood pressure below 130/80 mmHg reduces stress on grafts.

Regular Monitoring and Check-Ups

1. Patients with symptoms (chest pain, fatigue, breathlessness) should undergo stress tests or heart scans.
2. CT coronary angiography helps assess graft health without invasive procedures.

What if a Graft Gets Blocked Again?

Despite optimal medical therapy, a vein graft may get blocked again. Treatment depends on the patient's symptoms, severity of reduced blood flow and extent of graft obstruction.

Angioplasty and Stents (Percutaneous Coronary Intervention)

If only a small part of the graft is blocked, doctors may use balloon angioplasty and stents to open it.

Repeat Bypass Surgery

This surgery is rarely done because it carries higher surgical risks.

Intensified Medication Therapy

Higher doses of statins and stronger blood thinners may help keep partially blocked grafts open.

Key Research Studies Supporting Treatment

1. The PREVENT IV trial showed that many vein grafts fail in the first year post-CABG, highlighting the importance of strong blood-thinning therapy.[3]
2. The SYNTAX trial compared CABG and angioplasty, proving that medical therapy is essential for long-term graft survival.[4]
3. The REDUCE-IT study found that adding omega-3 fatty acids to statins reduces heart-related complications post-CABG.[5]

Educating Patients: Ensuring Long-Term Success

Medication Adherence

Many patients stop taking their medications too soon, increasing their risk of graft failure. Doctors should emphasise that lifelong medication use is critical.

Recognising Symptoms of Graft Failure

Patients should seek medical help if they experience chest pain, shortness of breath or unusual fatigue.

Cardiac Rehabilitation

Supervised exercise and counselling programmes help patients recover faster and stay committed to lifestyle changes.

The Learning

The success of bypass surgery, particularly with vein grafts, depends on not just the operation itself but on long-term care, medications and lifestyle changes. Vein grafts have a *higher failure rate* than arterial grafts, but proper use of blood thinners, statins and heart-protective drugs can greatly improve their survival. Patients must stay vigilant, follow prescribed treatments and work closely with their doctors to ensure long-lasting heart health and a better quality of life.

> The 'Widowmaker' artery is real. A blockage in the left anterior descending artery is deadly because it supplies a large part of the heart.

39

Understanding Pericardial Effusion

A THIRTY-FIVE-YEAR-OLD PATIENT presents with fever, progressive difficulty breathing, weight loss and some fluid around the heart, as seen on echocardiography. These symptoms suggest chronic issues with the pericardium (the heart's protective lining), which could be caused by infections, autoimmune disorders, cancer or metabolic problems. The severity of pericardial effusion, the fluid around the heart, can vary from mild to life-threatening. Hence, a detailed approach is needed for diagnosis and care.

Causes of Pericardial Effusion

Infectious Reasons

1. Viral infections: Common culprits include viruses like Coxsackievirus and the flu.
2. Tuberculosis: Often seen in regions where tuberculosis is prevalent, this can lead to weight loss and other system-wide symptoms.
3. Bacterial infections: They usually occur after pneumonia or blood infections.
4. Fungal infections: These infections are more common in people with weakened immune systems.

Cancer-Related Fluid

1. Spread of cancer (especially lung or breast cancer)
2. Pericardial tumours (rare but can be primary cancers like mesothelioma)

Autoimmune and Inflammatory Conditions

1. Systemic lupus erythematosus: It is characterised by fever and fluid accumulation.
2. Rheumatoid arthritis and systemic sclerosis: These can cause ongoing fluid accumulation.

Metabolic Issues

1. Kidney disease: It can lead to fluid build-up due to uraemia.
2. Hypothyroidism: This condition can also result in slow fluid accumulation.

Post-Cardiac Injury Syndromes

1. Dressler syndrome: Fluid may collect around the heart after a heart attack.
2. Post-surgery or injury: This often results in effusion.

Other Factors

1. Idiopathic effusion: No clear cause can be found, often determined by exclusion.
2. Radiation therapy: It can trigger inflammation and fluid build-up around the heart.

Recognising Symptoms of Pericardial Effusion

Common Symptoms

1. General symptoms: Fever, tiredness and weight loss
2. Heart-related symptoms: Chest pain (usually sharp), difficulty breathing and feeling of racing heartbeats
3. Severe symptoms: Signs of heart compression include shortness of breath, difficulty lying flat, erratic pulse and low blood pressure

Physical Examination Findings

1. Heart sounds might be distant or muffled.

2. Friction rub is a sound heard during inflammation of the pericardium.
3. Swollen neck veins indicates pressure on the heart from fluid build-up.

Diagnostic Process
1. Echocardiogram is a key test that confirms the presence of fluid and assesses severity. It can also show if the heart is under strain.
2. Lab tests
   a. Inflammation markers: High levels suggest underlying inflammation.
   b. Blood cultures: They are needed if bacteria are suspected.
   c. Autoimmune tests: Conditions like lupus or rheumatoid arthritis can be identified.
   d. Tuberculosis tests: Skin tests and sputum tests are included.
3. Fluid drainage: Pericardiocentesis is sometimes required for significant fluid or suspected infections/malignancies. The fluid is analysed for diagnosis.
4. Imaging techniques
   a. Chest X-ray can show heart enlargement in cases of significant effusion.
   b. CT/MRI scans are helpful in assessing thickening around the heart or associated tumours.

Managing Pericardial Effusion

The general approach is to treat the underlying cause and alleviate symptoms to avoid serious complications like heart compression. Targeted treatments are based on the cause.

Infectious Effusions

Viral Pericarditis

Medications such as nonsteroidal anti-inflammatory drugs (for example, ibuprofen) are given to reduce inflammation. Colchicine may help prevent recurrence. Corticosteroids are prescribed for severe cases only.

Tuberculous Pericarditis

Long-term anti-tuberculosis treatment is necessary. Corticosteroids are given for large effusions or where there is a risk of complications.

Bacterial Pericarditis

Broad-spectrum antibiotics can be given while waiting for culturing results. Drainage procedures must be done if necessary.

Fungal Pericarditis

Treatment is with antifungal medications along with fluid removal.

Malignant Effusion

1. Fluid drainage for relief: Procedures like therapeutic pericardiocentesis or a pericardial window can help relieve symptoms by removing excess fluid from around the heart.
2. Intrapericardial chemotherapy and radiotherapy: Sometimes, direct chemotherapy (like Cisplatin) or radiation treatment is used to target cancer cells in the fluid around the heart.
3. Systemic cancer treatment: Additional treatments depend on the type and stage of the cancer affecting the patient.

Autoimmune and Inflammatory Causes

Pericarditis from Systemic Lupus Erythematosus

1. Corticosteroids: High doses (for example, prednisone at 1 mg/kg per day) are used to reduce inflammation.
2. Immunosuppressants: Medications like azathioprine and mycophenolate are given for severe cases that don't respond to corticosteroids.

Pericarditis from Rheumatoid Arthritis

1. Pain relief: Nonsteroidal anti-inflammatory drugs and corticosteroids are recommended for treating acute fluid build-up.
2. Long-term control: Medications like methotrexate or biologics are used to manage the underlying disease.

Metabolic Causes

Uraemic Pericarditis

1. Intensive dialysis: An increased frequency of dialysis can help manage symptoms.
2. Pain relief: Nonsteroidal anti-inflammatory drugs can provide relief but should be used carefully in patients with kidney issues.
3. Fluid drainage: Pericardiocentesis might be needed if symptoms persist.

Hypothyroid Pericarditis

Thyroid treatment: Hormone replacement therapy with Levothyroxine helps manage this condition.

Drainage Procedures

1. Pericardiocentesis is a process to remove excess fluid from the pericardium, the sac surrounding the heart. This procedure is performed for large fluid build-up or if there are signs of heart strain caused by the fluid. Complications may include bleeding, heart rhythm problems or a punctured lung.
2. Pericardial window surgery is recommended for patients with recurring fluid build-up or specific fluid pockets that need attention.

Follow-Up and Long-Term Care

Managing Recurring Effusions

Colchicine may be used for fluid build-ups of unknown cause or due to inflammation. Repeating drainage procedures or considering surgery for ongoing issues might be necessary.

Preventing Complications

Regular monitoring for constrictive pericarditis is crucial, which may include imaging and studies to check heart function.

Prognosis

1. Idiopathic and viral effusions: Generally, the outlook is excellent with proper treatment.
2. Malignant effusions: The prognosis varies depending on the stage of the underlying cancer and how well it responds to treatment.
3. Tuberculous and bacterial effusions: The prognosis improves significantly with early diagnosis and appropriate treatment.

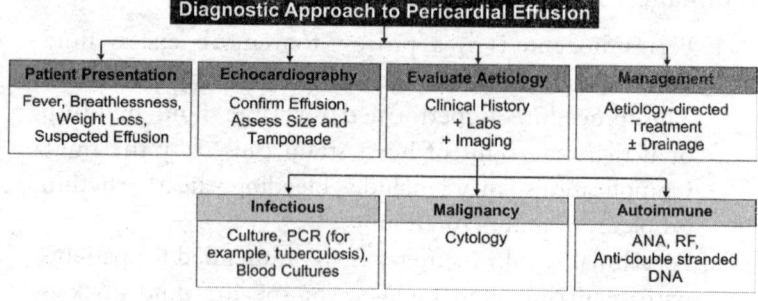

The Learning

Effectively managing moderate pericardial effusion involves a personalised approach based on the underlying cause. Quick diagnosis using echocardiograms, fluid analysis and advanced imaging is vital. Treatment tailored to specific causes – like anti-infective drugs, immunosuppressants or drainage procedures – ensures the best outcomes. Regular follow-up care is essential to watch for complications such as constrictive pericarditis or future fluid build-ups.

> Rapid fluid accumulation can cause significant heart problems and, in severe cases, can lead to heart failure or even death.

40

When Your Heart Skips a Beat – And Not in a Romantic Way

Understanding AFib

Atrial fibrillation, often called AFib, is a common heart condition that causes an irregular and sometimes very fast heartbeat. Think of your heart as a drummer in a band – when everything is working well, the rhythm is steady and predictable. But with AFib, it is like the drummer has lost their rhythm, making the beats unpredictable and sometimes too fast. This can make a person feel unwell and increases the risk of serious health problems, such as stroke.

This chapter will walk you through the signs and symptoms of AFib, how it is diagnosed, the different ways to treat it and how a special procedure can help prevent strokes in some patients.

Signs and Symptoms of AFib

Some people don't have any noticeable symptoms, which makes AFib tricky to diagnose without regular health check-ups. Here are some common signs:

1. Palpitations: You might feel like your heart is pounding, skipping beats or beating too fast.
2. Fatigue: Everyday tasks may leave you feeling exhausted.
3. Shortness of breath: You may struggle to catch your breath, especially when active or lying down.
4. Dizziness or light-headedness: Some people feel unsteady, like they might faint.

5. Chest discomfort: A feeling of tightness or mild pain may be felt in the chest.
6. Less stamina for exercise: Physical activities may feel more difficult than usual.

Diagnosis of AFib

Since AFib affects the heart's rhythm, the best way to detect it is by recording how the heart beats. Doctors use a few different tools to confirm AFib.

ECG

An ECG is the primary tool for diagnosing AFib. If there is a presence of AFib, then this test will show:

1. an *irregular rhythm* instead of a steady heartbeat,
2. absence of P waves (lack of *normal* electrical signals from the heart's upper chambers) and
3. fibrillatory waves (tiny, wavy lines that indicate disorganised heart activity).

These findings confirm the presence of AFib and help guide further management.

Echocardiography

It helps doctors see the following:

1. Chamber size and function: Assessment of atrial and ventricular dimensions and performance
2. Valvular abnormalities: Detection of any issues with heart valves
3. Thrombus formation: Identification of blood clots, particularly in the left atrial appendage

This imaging modality is crucial for evaluating structural heart disease and potential complications associated with AFib.

Treatment of AFib

AFib treatment aims to help patients feel better and reduce the risk of complications, like stroke. There are three main ways doctors manage AFib.

Controlling the Heart Rate

Instead of trying to fix the irregular rhythm, some treatments focus on keeping the heart from beating too fast. Common medicines include:

1. beta-blockers (for example, metoprolol) to slow the heart rate,
2. calcium channel blockers (for example, diltiazem) to help regulate the heartbeat and
3. digoxin, which is used in certain cases to slow the heart rate.

Restoring a Normal Rhythm

If the goal is to get the heart back into a normal rhythm, doctors may recommend:

1. antiarrhythmic medications (special drugs to stabilise the heartbeat),
2. electrical cardioversion (a controlled electric shock that resets the heart's rhythm) and
3. catheter ablation (a procedure where a thin tube is inserted into the heart to find and destroy the small areas causing the irregular beats)

Preventing Blood Clots and Strokes

When the heart beats irregularly, blood can pool and form clots, which can travel to the brain and cause a stroke. To lower this risk, doctors prescribe blood thinners such as warfarin, an older blood thinner that requires regular blood tests, and direct oral anticoagulants (for example, dabigatran, rivaroxaban, apixaban). The choice of anticoagulant depends on individual risk factors, bleeding risk and patient preferences.

Left Atrial Appendage Occlusion for Stroke Prevention

The left atrial appendage is a small, ear-shaped sac in the left atrium where blood clots commonly form in AFib patients. Occluding this appendage can reduce stroke risk, especially in patients who cannot tolerate long-term anticoagulation.

How Does the Procedure Work?

This is a minimally invasive procedure done through a small cut in the groin. A catheter is guided to the heart to place a tiny device inside the left atrial appendage, blocking blood from entering. Transoesophageal echocardiography and fluoroscopy are used to ensure accurate placement. This prevents clot formation and lowers stroke risk.

Why Do Some Patients Choose Left Atrial Appendage Occlusion?

1. It reduces stroke risk without the need for lifelong blood thinners.
2. It is a good option for patients who have a high risk of bleeding from blood thinners.
3. The procedure has risks, such as bleeding or device complications, but for some patients, the benefits outweigh these concerns.

Patient selection for this procedure should involve a thorough evaluation of risks and benefits, considering individual patient factors and preferences.

The Learning

AFib is a prevalent arrhythmia with significant health implications, including an increased risk of stroke. Recognising its signs and symptoms, utilising diagnostic tools like ECG and echocardiography and implementing appropriate treatment strategies are essential for effective management. The good news is that doctors have several ways to manage AFib, from medications to procedures that regulate heart rhythm and prevent blood clots.

For patients unsuitable for long-term anticoagulation, left atrial appendage occlusion offers an alternative strategy to reduce the risk of stroke associated with AFib.

If you or a loved one experiences symptoms like a racing heart, dizziness or fatigue, it is essential to seek medical advice. With the right treatment and lifestyle adjustments, people with AFib can live full and active lives. Understanding AFib is the first step towards managing it well, and now you have a clearer picture of what it means, how it is diagnosed and the available treatments.

---

50 per cent of heart attacks happen in people with 'normal' cholesterol. That is why screening for inflammation (high-sensitivity C-reactive protein), lipoprotein(a) and genetics is important.

41

Decoding Coronary Angiography: Why It Matters

CORONARY ANGIOGRAPHY IS A medical test that helps doctors see the blood vessels of the heart. It is used to check if there are any blockages or narrowing in these vessels, which can lead to heart problems. This test is especially useful for people who have chest pain, heart disease or other symptoms related to heart health.

Types of Coronary Angiography

There are different ways to perform coronary angiography, each with its own advantages.

Invasive Coronary Angiography

This is the most commonly used method. A catheter is inserted into a blood vessel and guided to the heart. A special contrast dye is then injected, and X-ray images are taken to see how blood is flowing through the arteries. It provides detailed visualisation of the coronary anatomy and is considered the gold standard for diagnosing coronary artery disease.

CT Coronary Angiography

This is a non-invasive imaging technique that uses CT scanning to visualise the coronary arteries. It is mostly used for people who have a lower risk of heart disease and helps rule out serious blockages.

Magnetic Resonance Angiography

This is another non-invasive method that uses MRI to visualise blood vessels. While less commonly used for coronary arteries due to lower spatial resolution, it can be beneficial in specific clinical scenarios.

When Is Coronary Angiography Needed?

Doctors recommend this test in the following situations:

1. Checking for heart blockages: If you have chest pain or symptoms of angina, this test helps determine if your arteries are blocked. This test helps in diagnosing obstructive coronary artery disease.
2. Acute coronary syndromes: If someone is having a heart attack or severe chest pain, angiography helps doctors decide if urgent treatment is needed.
3. Unclear stress test results: If previous tests show unclear or suspicious results, this test provides a clearer picture.
4. Evaluation before heart surgery: If a person needs heart valve surgery, doctors use angiography to plan the procedure.
5. Unexplained chest pain: If other tests don't explain chest pain, this test helps find the cause.

Preparation for Coronary Angiography

Before undergoing coronary angiography, patients should keep the following in mind:

1. Medical history: Inform your doctor about any medications, allergies (especially to iodine or contrast dye) or existing health conditions.
2. Fasting: You will need to avoid eating for at least 6 hours before the test, though drinking clear liquids may be allowed until 2 hours before.

3. Medication adjustments: Some medications, especially blood thinners or diabetes drugs, may need to be adjusted before the test.
4. Pre-test check-ups: Blood tests, ECG (heart test) and other checks might be done to ensure you're fit for the procedure.
5. Consent: Doctors will explain the test, including risks and benefits, and ask you to sign a consent form.

During the Procedure

1. Setting: The test is done in a special hospital room called a catheterisation lab (cath lab).
2. Anaesthesia: A small area in your wrist or groin is numbed with local anaesthesia.
3. Catheter placement: A thin tube is inserted into an artery and carefully moved towards the heart.
4. Contrast dye injection: A contrast dye is injected to make the arteries visible on X-ray images.
5. Monitoring: Your heart rate, blood pressure and oxygen levels will be checked throughout.

The procedure usually takes about 30–60 minutes. If a blockage is found, doctors may decide to open it up immediately using a balloon (angioplasty) or place a stent to keep the artery open.

After the Procedure

1. Recovery: You will rest in a recovery area for a few hours.
2. Sheath removal: The tube is removed, and pressure is applied to stop/prevent bleeding.
3. Monitoring: Nurses will keep an eye on your heart rate, blood pressure and the site where the catheter was inserted.
4. Activity limitations: Avoid heavy lifting and strenuous activities for a few days.

5. Drinking water: This helps flush out the contrast dye from your body.
  6. Medication instructions: Your doctor will tell you when to resume your regular medications.

Possible Risks and Complications

While the test is generally safe, there are some risks to be aware of:

  1. Bruising or bleeding is common at the insertion site but usually mild.
  2. Some people may have allergic reactions to the contrast dye.
  3. Temporary irregular heart rhythms can occur.
  4. The dye can sometimes affect kidney function, especially in people with kidney disease.
  5. Though rare, there's a small risk of infection at the catheter site.
  6. Very rarely, serious complications such as a heart attack or stroke can occur during the procedure.

After the test, your doctor will review the images and discuss the findings with you. Based on the results, they may recommend lifestyle changes, medications or further procedures if needed.

The Learning

Coronary angiography is an important test that helps diagnose and manage heart disease. Knowing what to expect before, during and after the procedure can help ease concerns and ensure a smooth experience. Whether done through traditional methods or modern imaging techniques, the goal remains the same – to keep your heart healthy and functioning well. CT coronary angiography is a great tool for ruling out heart disease, especially in younger individuals without risk factors. However, it may not be as effective for older adults with existing conditions like diabetes or smoking history. In such cases, it can sometimes create more confusion rather than providing a clear answer.

If you have concerns about your heart health, speak to your doctor about whether this test is right for you!

> 'Angioplasty with stenting does not treat the underlying causes of blockages in your arteries.'
>
> Mayo Clinic[1]

Notes

Chapter 1 Ticking Time Bomb: How One Man's Denial Cost Him Everything

1. 'The Blood Flow Through the Heart?', Cleveland Clinic. Available online: https://my.clevelandclinic.org/health/articles/17060-how-does-the-blood-flow-through-your-heart

Chapter 2 A Race Against Time: Sandhya's Battle for Every Breath

1. '5 Heart Facts That May Surprise You', Johns Hopkins Medicine. Available online: https://www.hopkinsmedicine.org/health/wellness-and-prevention/5-heart-facts-that-may-surprise-you

Chapter 3 Defying the Unthinkable: Power Athlete Dhriti's Hidden Battle

1. 'Hypertension', World Health Organization. Available online: https://www.who.int/news-room/fact-sheets/detail/hypertension

Chapter 4 Shattered Rhythm: The Unseen Battle Behind the Mic

1. 'Anxiety and Heart Disease', Johns Hopkins Medicine. Available online: https://www.hopkinsmedicine.org/health/conditions-and-diseases/anxiety-and-heart-disease

Chapter 5 Too Young to Fall: The Catastrophic Heartbreak

1. Cleveland Clinic, 'Heart Valves'. Available online: https://my.clevelandclinic.org/health/body/17067-heart-valves

Chapter 6 The Poisoned Cure

1. Editorial Staff, 'Effects of Alcoholism on Families and Close Friends', Alcohol.org, 25 October 2022. Available online: https://alcohol.org/faq/problems-associated-with-alcoholism/

Chapter 7 Like Father, Like Son: A Fight Against Recurrence

1. Gunjan K. Ghodeshwar, Amol Dube and Deepa Khobragade, 'Impact of Lifestyle Modifications on Cardiovascular Health: A Narrative Review', *Cureus*, 15 (7): e42616. DOI 10.7759/cureus.42616. Available online: https://assets.cureus.com/uploads/review_article/pdf/172900/20230827-13768-ce23up.pdf

Chapter 8 The Fallen Star: Heartbreak on the Field

1. 'Why Indians?/ Why South Asians?', Indian Heart Association. Available online: https://indianheartassociation.org/why-indians-why-south-asians/

Chapter 9 Pregnancy and the Heart

1. 'South Asian Women and Heart Disease', Indian Heart Association. Available online: https://indianheartassociation.org/south-asian-women-and-heart-disease/

Chapter 10 Beyond the Reps: Gym and Sudden Cardiac Deaths

1. Personal communication with Dr Sharma.

Chapter 15 Heart Attack After Surgery

1. Anthony A. Bavry, 'Perioperative Ischemic Evaluation 2 – POISE-2', American College of Cardiology, 14 November 2017. Available online: https://www.acc.org/Latest-in-Cardiology/Clinical-Trials/2014/05/03/19/28/POISE-2
2. Annemarie Thompson et al., '2024 AHA/ACC/ACS/ASNC/HRS/SCA/SCCT/SCMR/SVM Guideline for Perioperative Cardiovascular Management for Noncardiac Surgery: A Report of the American College of Cardiology/American Heart Association Joint Committee on Clinical Practice Guidelines', Citation,

150 (9). Available online: https://www.ahajournals.org/doi/10.1161/CIR.0000000000001285#:~:text=Take%2DHome%20Messages-,1.,real%20consequences%20for%20affected%20patients

CHAPTER 16 BLUE BABIES AND AN ASYMPTOMATIC ADULT

1. '5 Must-Know Facts about Congenital Heart Disease in Children: CHD Stats and What You Can Do', Children's HeartLink, 17 February 2025. Available online: https://childrensheartlink.org/congenital-heart-disease-facts/

CHAPTER 18 BEYOND SNORING: A SCARY WAKE-UP CALL

1. Imre Janszky et al., 'Heavy Snoring Is a Risk Factor for Case Fatality and Poor Short-term Prognosis After a First Acute Myocardial Infarction', *Sleep*, 31(6): 801–07. doi: 10.1093/sleep/31.6.801. Available online: https://pmc.ncbi.nlm.nih.gov/articles/PMC2442412/#:~:text=Heavy%20snoring%2C%20especially%20if%20regular,%2C%20stroke%2C%20or%20heart%20failure

CHAPTER 19 WOMEN AND HEART ATTACKS

1. 'Women & CVD', World Heart Foundation. Available online: https://world-heart-federation.org/what-we-do/women-cvd/

CHAPTER 20 RIGHT HEART FAILURE IN ALCOHOLIC LIVER DISEASE

1. 'Study Links Heavy Drinking to Increased Heart Disease Risk in Young Women', News Medical Life Sciences, 28 March 2024. Available online: https://www.news-medical.net/news/20240328/Study-links-heavy-drinking-to-increased-heart-disease-risk-in-young-women.aspx

CHAPTER 25 EXERCISE AND THE HEART

1. 'American Heart Association Recommendations for Physical Activity in Adults and Kids', American Heart Association. Available online: https://www.heart.org/en/healthy-living/fitness/fitness-basics/aha-recs-for-physical-activity-in-adults

CHAPTER 26 POLLUTION AND THE HEART

1. 'New Delhi Air Quality Index (AQI) | Air Pollution', AQI. Available online: https://www.aqi.in/us/dashboard/india/delhi/new-delhi; Eric Koons, 'Delhi Smog: A Look at the Crisis and Pathway to

Cleaner Skies', Climate Tracker Impacts Asia, 7 November 2024. Available online: https://www.climateimpactstracker.com/delhi-smog/

2. 'Mumbai Particulate Matter (PM2.5) Level', AQI. Available online: https://www.aqi.in/us/dashboard/india/maharashtra/mumbai/pm; Rajendra Tatu Nanavare, 'Impact of Air Pollution on Respiratory Health: A Case Study in Mumbai, India', *International Journal of Medical and Health Research*, 1 (1): 52–56. Available online: https://www.medicalsciencejournal.com/assets/archives/2024/vol10issue1/10009.pdf

3. 'Kolkata Particulate Matter (PM2.5) Level', AQI. Available online: https://www.aqi.in/us/dashboard/india/west-bengal/kolkata/pm; J. Karmakar, 'Assessing Human Health Risks from Particulate Matter Pollution: A Study of PM2.5 in the Kolkata Metropolitan Area', *Urban Studies*, 17 (4): 11–26. Available online: https://www.researchgate.net/publication/388452350_Assessing_Human_Health_Risks_from_Particulate_Matter_Pollution_A_Study_of_PM25_in_the_Kolkata_Metropolitan_Area

4. 'Chennai Particulate Matter (PM2.5) Level', AQI. Available online: https://www.aqi.in/us/dashboard/india/tamil-nadu/chennai/pm; P. Mangaraj, S.K. Sahu, G. Beig, A. Mishra and S. Sharma, 'What Makes the Indian Megacity Chennai's Air Unhealthy? - A Bottom-up Approach to Understand the Sources of Air Pollutants', *Aerosol and Air Quality Research*, 24 (9). Available online: https://aaqr.org/articles/aaqr-24-03-oa-0089

5. 'Bangalore Particulate Matter (PM2.5) Level', AQI. Available online: https://www.aqi.in/us/dashboard/india/karnataka/bangalore/pm; Prajwal Bhatt, 'B'luru's Air Pollution Contributing to Heart Diseases? Study Finds Drivers Are at Risk', The News Minute, 1 October 2019. Available online: https://www.thenewsminute.com/karnataka/blurus-air-pollution-contributing-heart-diseases-study-finds-drivers-are-risk-109819

Chapter 27 Food and Heart Health

1. Susan Hewlings, 'Coconuts and Health: Different Chain Lengths of Saturated Fats Require Different Consideration', *Journal of Cardiovascular Development and Disease*, 7 (4): 59. 17 December 2020. https://doi.org/10.3390/jcdd7040059. Available online: https://www.mdpi.com/2308-3425/7/4/59

Chapter 29 Can Heart Diseases Be Reversed?

1. 'Can We Reduce Plaque Buildup in Arteries?', Harvard Health Publishing, 4 August 2023. Available online: https://www.health.harvard.edu/heart-health/can-we-reduce-vascular-plaque-buildup
2. 'Undo It with Ornish', Healthways. Available online: https://www.uclahealth.org/sites/default/files/documents/Ornish_LiteratureReview.pdf?f=90b7156a

Chapter 32 Breathing and Meditation

1. A.A. Tseng, 'Scientific Evidence of Health Benefits by Practicing Mantra Meditation: Narrative Review', *International Journal of Yoga*, 15 (2):89–95. doi: 10.4103/ijoy.ijoy_53_22. Available online: https://pmc.ncbi.nlm.nih.gov/articles/PMC9623891/

Chapter 34 Varicose Veins

1. Lisa Catanese, 'Pulmonary Embolism: Symptoms, Causes, Risk Factors, and Treatment', Harvard Health Publishing, 21 December 2023. Available online: https://www.health.harvard.edu/diseases-and-conditions/pulmonary-embolism-symptoms-causes-risk-factors-and-treatment

Chapter 35 Valvular Heart Disease

1. N. Ktenopoulos et al., 'Emerging Transcatheter Therapies for Valvular Heart Disease: Focus on Mitral and Tricuspid Valve Procedures', *Life* (Basel), 14 (7): 842. doi: 10.3390/life14070842. Available online: https://pmc.ncbi.nlm.nih.gov/articles/PMC11277877/

Chapter 36 Mending the Holes in the Heart: Device Closure Versus Surgery

1. 'Why South Asians?', Indian Heart Association. Available online: https://indianheartassociation.org/why-indians-why-south-asians/overview/#:~:text=Demographic%20data%20indicate%20that%20the,demographics%2C%20often%20without%20prior%20warning

Chapter 37 Chest Pain

1. It refers to a type of heart attack where there is a partial blockage of a coronary artery, leading to reduced blood flow and oxygen to the heart muscle, but without specific ST-segment elevation on an ECG.

Chapter 38 Coronary Artery Bypass Surgery

1. Alexander Kulik et al., 'Secondary Prevention After Coronary Artery Bypass Graft Surgery: A Scientific Statement from the American Heart Association', *Circulation*, 131 (10). Available online: https://www.ahajournals.org/doi/10.1161/cir.0000000000000182; C.N. Hess et al., 'Saphenous Vein Graft Failure after Coronary Artery Bypass Surgery: Insights from PREVENT IV', *Circulation*, 130 (17): 1445–51. doi: 10.1161/CIRCULATIONAHA.113.008193. Available online: https://pmc.ncbi.nlm.nih.gov/articles/PMC4206593/#:~:text=Data%20source%20and%20patient%20population&text=Briefly%2C%20PREVENT%20IV%20was%20a,100%20sites%20(Figure%201)
2. Caroline Brigan, 'Statins Reduce Deaths from Heart Disease by 28 Per Cent, Says Longest Ever Study', Imperial, 6 September 2017. Available online: https://www.imperial.ac.uk/news/181453/statins-reduce-deaths-from-heart-disease/
3. Hess et al., 'Saphenous Vein Graft Failure'.
4. Patrick W. Serruys et al., 'Percutaneous Coronary Intervention versus Coronary-Artery Bypass Grafting for Severe Coronary Artery Disease', *New England Journal of Medicine*, 360 (10): 961–72. Available online: https://www.nejm.org/doi/full/10.1056/NEJMoa0804626
5. Deepak Bhatt, 'Reduction of Cardiovascular Events with Icosapent Ethyl–Intervention Trial – REDUCE-IT', American College of Cardiology, 2022. Available online: https://www.acc.org/Latest-in-Cardiology/Clinical-Trials/2018/11/08/22/48/REDUCE-IT

Chapter 41 Decoding Coronary Angiography: Why It Matters

1. 'Coronary Angioplasty and Stents', Mayo Clinic. Available online: https://www.mayoclinic.org/tests-procedures/coronary-angioplasty/about/pac-20384761

About the Authors

Dr Amit Bhushan Sharma is an award-winning cardiologist and director and head of cardiology at Paras Hospital, Gurugram. A fellow of the European Society of Cardiology and the Society for Cardiovascular Angiography and Interventions, he has twice been recognised as the best cardiology consultant in Delhi-NCR.

With over two decades of experience at leading hospitals, including Artemis and Apollo, Dr Sharma combines cutting-edge medical expertise with a deep belief in preventive heart care. As the co-founder and president of the Training Academy of Cardiac and Vascular Interventions, he trains young doctors and champions greater awareness of heart health for every age and lifestyle.

Former content strategist and now screen club director with GurgaonMoms, **Ambika Rikhye** – author of *Mirage* (2014) and co-author of *Bundle of Joy* (published by Bloomsbury in 2024) – writes with warmth and wit, leaving readers moved, inspired and unable to forget the worlds she creates through her writing.